The Lazy Keto

Gourmet

Includes:
* 50 low-carb, high-fat recipes
* No Artificial Sweeteners
* My Daily Menus
* Weight Loss Tips

Nissa Graun

From

Eating Fat is the New Skinny

Dedication:

This book is dedicated to my husband, Jason, who will never read this book because I already cook these delicious recipes for him.

Also to my kids, Charlie and Joey, who stopped jumping on me for a few minutes each day while I put this book together.

Contents

Introduction:

The Lazy Keto Gourmet has humble beginnings. Humble as in I grew up a latchkey kid who dipped smushed up bread into ketchup for lunch. Obviously that type of lunch was not sustainable, so I taught myself how to cook the basics - frozen pizzas, boxed mac & cheese, Steak-Ums and Carl Budding sandwiches on Wonder Bread. Actually, I don't think my single parent household could afford Wonder Bread, although we definitely had a few packages of Carl Budding at all times. Hopefully that makes you cringe just as much as I do now.

I grew up surrounded by fast food and processed junk. I tried to eat as much as I could as quickly as I could before my older brothers scarfed it all down. I developed an early addiction to fast food. McDonalds, Burger King, White Castle, Arbys...you name it, I had a favorite meal at that establishment. I could never understand why people would drool over a succulent home cooked meal when they could indulge in a McDouble for only 99 cents! That may be because my mom worked a lot. She worked very hard to provide for her three kids, so I might go so far as to say her kitchen skills were at times lacking.

This one time she made hamburgers and mixed the ground beef with oatmeal. Oatmeal burgers are even worse than they sound. Sorry mom. She is going to kill me for bringing that up again. She also had a penchant for throwing a bunch of leftovers together for a "new casserole" dinner. Who wouldn't prefer to hit up the drive thru for a #1 with a Diet Coke?

When I hit my early teens, I noticed my weight on an upward trajectory. All I knew about weight loss at the time was to watch less *Sally Jessy Raphael* (because what twelve year old isn't obsessed with daytime tv?) and exercise more. Then I went to see a registered dietitian.

During my eighth grade cheerleading physical, it was noted that my weight and cholesterol levels were on the rise. The dietitian explained these issues at an early age were due to my love of fast food and too many fat grams. She told me to cut portions of potato chips and fries in half, add low calorie drinks like diet soda and avoid fatty foods like red meat, butter and eggs. Ms. Dietitian suggested I fill up on the bottom foods listed on the food pyramid, which she dutifully pointed out on the handy dandy print out she sent home with me.

Low-fat was the craze of the decade and it is what I was taught would make me healthy. I tried hard to follow the dietitian's advice and developed a strong taste for Cocoa Pebbles in skim milk, spaghetti with marinara and boxed low calorie convenience foods. Basically anything described as a low-fat pizza meal was my favorite. Food marketers convinced me a low calorie Lean Cuisine with a diet soda was the healthy choice. In fact, Healthy Choice is an actual name of a brand I commonly purchased. Somehow I convinced myself that cardboard pizzas with tasteless low-fat cheese was a suitable meal. I told myself if I ate microwaved convenience foods for most meals, I would magically be thin. Those meals were already portioned out, which made it easy to add up daily calories.

Right...because that is how we are taught to lose weight. Counting calories is an absolute must in order to lose weight. Let me tell you, I counted calories for decades and I was damn good at it! At first I needed to carry around notebooks filled with serving sizes in order to tally up totals. As I honed my calorie counting craft, I could look at a meal and tell you the amount of calories it contained. I can still quote calorie counts to this day. There is so much useless calorie information filling up my head. I would like to hit Control + Alt + Delete to reset since I now understand this all means very little on a quest to optimal health.

I can't blame yo-yoing weight since my teenage years on lack of knowledge regarding cutting carbs either. I knew all about low-carb diets for almost as long as I have been trying to lose weight. The first time I attempted the Atkins diet was my freshman year in college. Since I went to a local community college for the first two years in order to stay close to a boyfriend, I can't even blame the freshman 15 most students battle after months of indulgent trips to the buffet. I was battling the bulge for a good seven years by this point.

Thus began sporadic attempts of eating deli ham dipped in mayo and ordering extra mystery meat from Taco Bell since I would not be partaking in the protective shells. This seemed to be a wonderful lifestyle filled with unlimited bacon, steak and cheese. Every attempt I made, this was the best diet on the planet; at least for the first few weeks. At that point I could no longer stomach one more hamburger patty with no bun, no ketchup and no sides of fun!

To be honest, I could not let go of calorie counting. Even when I made another low-carb attempt, most of the time I dipped lean chicken breasts into low-fat mayo. There were hardly any carbs, so I thought I had it right. Most diet plans I sought out told me to aim for 1200 - 1300 calories for a female of my height who desired weight loss. I zeroed in on that total for years. Sometimes I hit it daily for months and lost a few pounds. Other times I found myself gorging on two Big Mac Meals with a Diet Coke because I felt so horrible from stomping my metabolism into the ground. I needed nourishment quick! Once again I stopped my latest low-carb attempt and the weight came back twice as fast as it left.

At the time I did not know I was stomping my metabolism into the ground. That's what I was told was necessary in order to hit my goal. I also did not know not a single item at McDonald's actually constitutes nourishment. For many years after my first attempt at a low-carb diet, I tried time and again to ride the low-carb train. I ordered those McDoubles and whipped the bun off every time. I mixed these sad attempts in with stints at Weight Watchers, Jenny Craig and LA Weight Loss. I lost and regained the same twenty to fifty pounds year after year for more than 20 years.

I also became an over-exerciser at a young age. Instead of zoning out to daytime talk shows, I ran in place in my bedroom while blasting Bon Jovi. A really cool network arrived on the scene called the *Cable Fit Club*. It starred Jake from Body by Jake and Tami Lee Webb. I didn't know who these fitness gurus were - but they were in shape and the workouts were free. I spent many afternoons following along to step aerobics on cruise ships while stationed in my tiny bedroom, stumbling over a teal styrofoam step.

While we are on this subject, am I the only person in the room who took full advantage of *Body Electric*? Look it up. I was twelve years old and following along to a show whose tagline is, "Aging is a fact of life, but you don't have to put out the welcome mat." Every young girl's dream, those free PBS shows that feature older ladies in leotards getting buff with low resistance weights.

I will say Margaret Richard was stacked. I will also say I worked with what I had back in the day. At home fitness has come a long way since the days of *Body Electric*.

The day I turned eighteen, I left free PBS shows behind since I was old enough to sign up for Bally Total Fitness. I finally got to workout with the big boys; except I typically stuck with the women in the cardio rooms. The weight rooms filled with buff bros were intimidating to say the least. I also had no clue what to do with those resistance machines and had very little energy leftover after my

60-90 minute cardio session. I spent a lot of my life on machines like elliptical trainers, stairmasters, stationary bikes and treadmills. That is what I considered exercise variety in those days.

Those were the beginnings of my "move more, eat less" roots. I moved a lot and ate very little for decades. The food marketers and fitness gurus convinced me eating "healthy" processed junk while spinning my wheels on stationary bikes for hours each day was the only path to optimal health. Throughout this twenty year duration, my health was poor and my belly bulge always hung over the sides of my jeans. I wrote an entire book about that journey: *My Big Fat Life Transformation* available on Amazon. Check it out to learn the full harrowing tale.

Let's Get Cooking

In 2013 I reached my highest weight ever after the birth of my first son. A 245 pound Nissa had no clue how to cook beyond preheating the oven and throwing in a pre-packaged convenience food. There were days I even screwed up those meals. Burnt yet still chewy boxed lasagna is not the treat it appears as shown on the box.

OK, so I knew how to make some of the basics. I made a mean taco meat and spaghetti meat sauce. I also cooked chicken breasts, but only the rubbery kind. Throughout most of my days spent yo-yoing back and forth on the scale, I ate out a lot. I lived in Chicago at the time and in the case you've never been, Chicago has really good takeout options. It's hard to settle for rubbery chicken when you know a beef with red sauce and fries is less than a ten minute drive away. Tasting those salty sticks of heaven was completely worth the 45 minutes I had to drive around in search of a parking spot.

Since I stayed at home with my son, it became difficult to sneak away for the takeout lunches I became accustomed to when I worked in office settings. Then there's my husband of just over a year. The man expected dinner some nights. Some of those nights he even expected me to cook that dinner. Gasp!

Throwing together a Hamburger Helper meal wasn't too big of a burden, but since we both wanted to take off some pounds, the boxed meals were out. I came across a book called *Kick Your Fat in the Nuts.* The book teaches you to eat less than 25 grams of carbs with meals, while also raising healthy fats. The author focuses on eating real food - not the kind that is fast, easy or cheap. Double gasp! So long french fries; we knew each other well.

I read the book a few times and took the corresponding 12 Week Online Fat Loss Course. I studied hard in order for all of this new knowledge to sink in. The book and the course work together to teach how to improve digestive malfunctions that could be holding someone back from losing weight and gaining optimal health. That is the book that brought me back kicking and screaming to low-carb diets.

After twenty years of struggle I no longer wanted any kind of diet, little lone a diet that took away my precious dinner rolls. I caved, but this time I stuck with it...like for a really long time. I followed the instructions in the book and the course and somehow low-carb diets became easy for me after many hardcore struggles with them in the past.

The biggest part of that was improving my digestion with natural supplements so my body could start to recognize other food as fuels beyond processed carbohydrates. For the first time in as long as I could remember, eating protein and fat together without half of my plate consisting of something starchy became normal. The cravings for highly processed junk foods started to disappear. This was all very new and exciting to me. There were years I subsisted junk carbs alone. Did I mention how sick and fat I was during those years? If you are living on only junk carbs and you too feel sick and fat, trust me when I tell you there is a connection.

Suddenly I was a brand new me! A friend could bring a box of donuts to my house and I would not even be tempted to snag the last Boston Creme since my body was filled up with the good stuff; all of the vitamins, healthy fats and proteins those donuts do not contain. In the past I would not call a person who brings donuts over while I am on a diet a friend at all, but this time it was easy not to want to poke her eyes out with my asparagus spears. I ate the asparagus spears instead and observed my friend's energy quickly crash and burn from the two sugar bombs she gobbled up in two minutes flat.

I completely skipped over the mention of asparagus because I was so excited to tell you how I no longer wanted what I previously considered sugary pillows of love. I taught myself how to cook real, whole foods like asparagus!

Well, actually not asparagus. The digestive supplements and consumption of real foods are excellent ways to train your brain to prefer the good stuff, but I still do not get the appeal of asparagus. I prefer normal smelling pee, thank you very much. I did learn to cook other real foods with nutrients my body requires to thrive. Not only did I learn to cook homemade meals, but my Google inspired experiments were delicious! Who knew foods without pretty pictures on boxes displaying photos of the end result could actually taste good?

That's how we arrived here. Since my mother's cooking methods were a fail, I had to use Google to teach myself to cook. The more I cooked real foods at home, the tastier my home cooked meals became. Practice really does make perfect. I tried several different low-carb cookbooks too, but I found myself spending far too much time tracking down exotic ingredients and figuring out the meanings of fancy terms like "fold in." While reading a cookbook, you probably expect the author to know things like that. I do now, but the first few recipes I had to fold ingredients into, I had no clue.

This brings me to an important point. I titled this book *The Lazy Keto Gourmet* because it is not filled with fancy cooking terms and methods novices do not understand. That's not how real people do this. My recipes are not filled with exotic ingredients you have to hit up five different stores to find. I'm a stay-at-home mom of small children. The less I have to leave my house, the better. That means many of the ingredients I use can be found in online marketplaces like Thrive Market.

If you are not currently ordering from Thrive Market, click the link on my website to check them out. You will even save 25% on your first order. They do have a yearly subscription fee which put me off at first. I wish I knew how convenient ordering is and how much money I would actually save for that convenience much sooner. I easily make up the cost of the membership in dark chocolate alone.

If you are more of a pro than most, don't judge me for my methods. There is enough mommy shaming in the world as it is. As I said, I knew nothing. I taught myself from scratch. The recipes I make are easy for the novice and taste better than most dishes I order from fancy restaurants on a rare date night out. I lick the bowl of practically every recipe I make. That has to mean something.

I know fancy, schmancy cooks would never admit to licking bowls either, but I'm just a stay-at-home mom, remember? Nothing fancy, schmancy about me. I lick bowls and I don't feel guilty about it because my recipes are filled with the delicious, healthy fats my body needs to thrive. There will be no healthy fats wasted in this household.

My recipes have also had more than 200,000 views in less than a year. For an unknown stay-at-home mom of littles who licks all of her fat bomb bowls, that's kind of a big deal. Like, I *need* to write a cookbook big deal. That's why we are here.

Another thing fancy-schmancy cooks do is use proper equipment like double boilers to melt chocolate. I try to buy as little kitchen equipment as I can since somehow all of our storage cabinets are already full. That means I melt chocolate on low heat in a saucepan instead of a double boiler. I don't exactly know how much space a double boiler would take up, but it is space we do not have and the saucepan works just fine. I make fat bombs at least three times per week, no double boiler required. If you want to use fancier cookware such as this, go for it! You are never limited to the scope of this book.

Let's Get Learning

On a different note, I have also learned a lot about how our bodies are supposed to function and how to take advantage of that with a low-carb, high-fat diet. In order to lose more than 100 pounds and end yo-yo diets for good, I *had* to learn a lot. Losing that amount of weight and maintaining the loss long term doesn't just happen. Education about your specific body is key to success. If I just gave you these high-fat recipes and let you out into the world all alone, you would suffer. You would be cold and alone and drown in a world of endless coconut oil and butter. In that respect I am going to teach along the way how to use these recipes to optimize your digestion and how not to get fat while eating a lot of fat.

This is a cookbook, so there is only so much I can teach in this book. I will do my best. If you are ready for even more learning and witty banter, you have several options available to you. I have a website - eatingfatisthenewskinny.com. My website has blogs, videos and recipes to help you along your low-carb, high-fat journey.

I constantly receive the question of how I had such great success when so many others struggle. With a four year old constantly shouting, "Hey mom, look at this!" and a two year old who only finds solace sitting on mommy's lap most days, I don't have time to start from scratch with every amazed person I meet. This is precisely the reason I wrote the book I mentioned earlier. I want to help people get started on their own path to low-carb, high-fat success, but I don't want to get bashed in the head by my flailing toddler when I look away for one moment to answer the same question again. The book is on Amazon and is called *My Big Fat Life Transformation* in case you read right past that mention. If you read it and love it, I would appreciate a book review to help spread the low-carb, high-fat love.

If you cannot get enough of these health knowledge nuggets and yearn to know even more, you, dear friend, are going to be successful. That is exactly my attitude with all of this fascinating health information. I want to know more and I want to know it all right now. For those over-achievers, I put together a six week course jam packed with information and motivation for a successful low-carb, high-fat life. My *Coach Me Course: Escape DIet Mentality and End Yo-Yo Diets Forever* is a full six weeks of daily emails, weekly videos and helpful guides. That's obviously way too much information to add to a cookbook, so take the course if you want to make this lifestyle easier.

As you can see, there are plenty of ways to learn beyond this book filled with delicious recipes, but let's start here. Try the easy recipes, read the helpful notes in between sections, and live a life filled with delicious foods that keep you healthy while helping you reach your goals. Easy peasy lemon squeezy.

Let's Get Started!
But First - A Few Important Notes

You may notice not a one of the recipes listed in this book contain macros. How the heck are you supposed to follow a diet based on macros without having macros specifically spelled out for you? This may cause you to ask the question, "Who is this magic woman who lost more than 150 pounds combined without knowing every last macro she shoved into her face?"

Magic woman I am not. Lazy with my food choices? Check!

I personally do not believe you need to know every last macro you shove into your mouth in order to be successful on a ketogenic diet. I left that sort of obsessiveness behind long ago along with counting points in my many stints of

Weight Watchers. These days I am much more relaxed about the food I eat. With this method, I have found much greater success and an easy lifestyle.

When I started out on my keto diet, I had a basic knowledge of approximate carb consumption and ate fat and protein until I felt satiated. On occasions I hit weight loss stalls, I double checked to make sure my protein was in check and my fat was high enough to maintain ketosis. I feel like that is the best way to succeed - not to obsess. You may be different, and that's cool.

If you absolutely must have macros, I will teach you how to fish. Download your favorite macro tracking app to your phone. Mine is Cronometer. Click on the button that lets you make a recipe. Add in all ingredients you use into the recipe builder; divide by the amount of servings in your recipe. Poof! Macros for days! Most of the apps will allow you to save your macro information for the next time you want to eat the same recipe.

Some of the recipes in this book do have macros listed on my website eatingfatisthenewskinny.com. Check the bottom of the corresponding recipe. Feel free to recalculate your own macros in the case your ingredients vary from mine.

One last thing before we start. I am not a doctor. Do not take anything written in this book as medical advice. It is just a cookbook written by a stay-at-home mom, after all. You can use what I have learned to expand your own knowledge, but if you are seeking medical advice do so only from the doctor you choose.

Lazy Keto Gourmet

Breakfasts

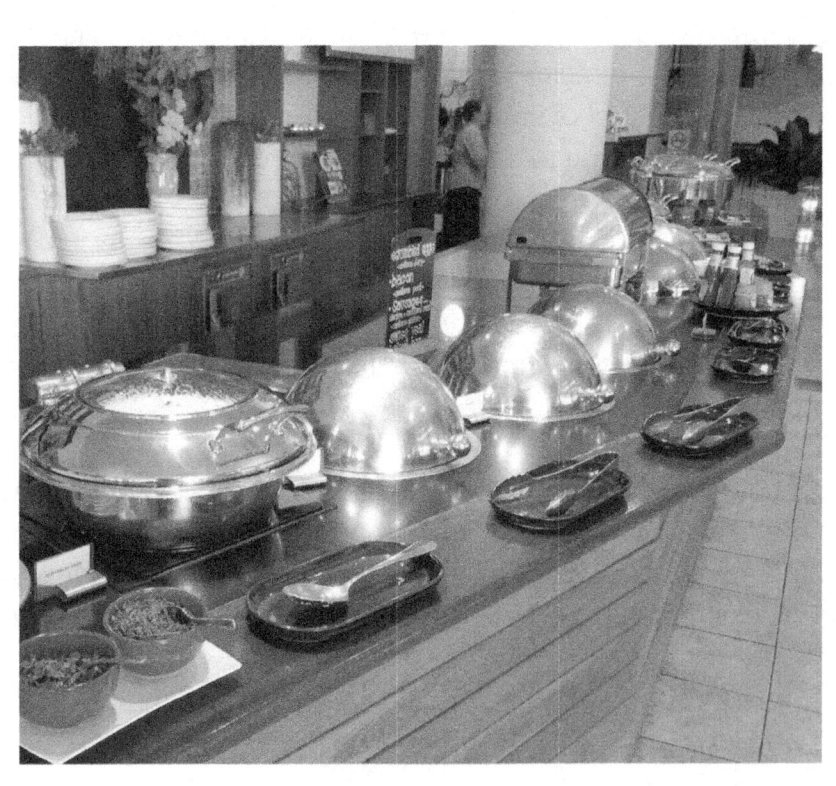

Break-Fast

Let's start with breakfast - the most important meal of the day.

I'm not 100% on board with that statement. I repeated it because it is catchy and a phrase most people parrot. Not everyone *needs* to eat breakfast just because everyone insists *you need* to eat breakfast. I don't; at least not in the traditional sense. I am in the best health of my life and maintain a healthy weight.

Quit listening to people who scream at you that you must eat all day, everyday in order to obtain a fast metabolism and healthy weight. Most of those people screaming at you are food marketers or people who work closely with food marketers. Many others follow blindly behind.

If your digestion is not on track, you probably don't even want to eat breakfast because your body is still dealing with the burden you gave it the night before. If that is the case for you, do not force yourself to eat a typical breakfast upon rising because that's what you are told to do in order to be healthy. That being said, if yours is a case of impaired digestion, start working on that. Who wants to eat foods your body views as toxins, only to have those foods rotting and fermenting in your stomach anyway? That is going to lead to gas pains, constipation, difficulty losing weight and a slew of other undesirable health conditions.

Most people reading this cookbook will eat breakfast at some point during the day. The word breakfast is derived from breaking your fast from the night before. Whether you eat it at 7 am or noon, it technically is still breakfast. If you want to eat bacon and eggs, cool! If you want to heat up marinated steak strips from the night before, that works too. Mix them together for steak and eggs if that floats your low-carb boat, but only if your digestion is on par because that is a heavy meal to digest.

Lazy Gourmet Eggs

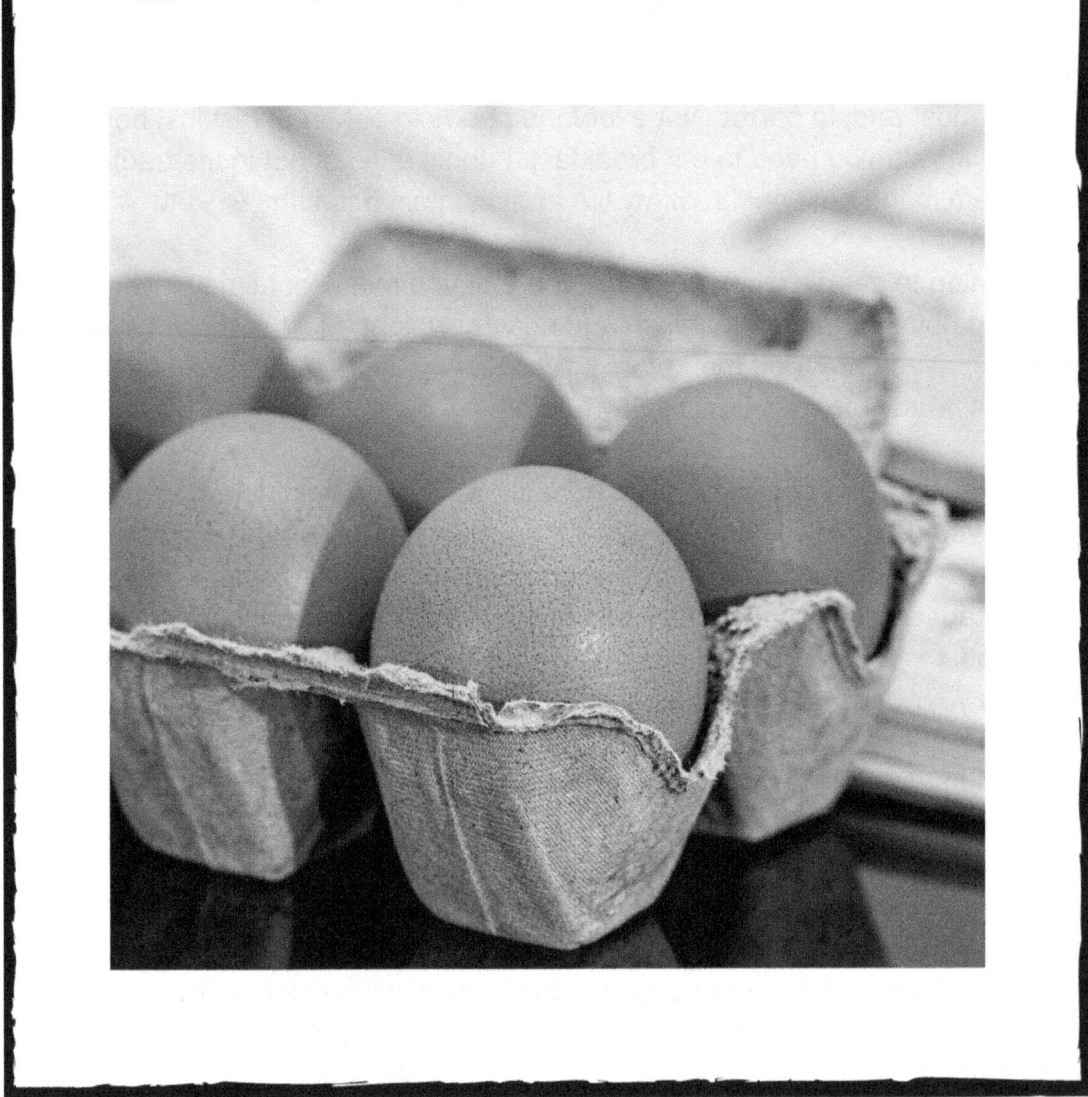

The Incredible Edible Egg

Let's talk eggs for a moment. Growing up I did not enjoy eggs at all. I rushed to the pancake section and doused those cakes with the sweetest syrup I could find. Mmmmm, syrupy cakes for breakfast. That's what our government promotes as a healthy start to our day.

Once I began low-carb, high-fat diets in my late teens, I realized eggs are pretty much the standard LCHF breakfast. Of course there was misinformation being pushed out in every direction. Even though I felt better when I ate eggs for breakfast, I still had nutrition authorities whispering in my ear, "High cholesterol! Too much fat! BUYER BEWARE!" To this day cereal lobbyists are still finding sneaky ways to promote high sugar cereals over what is possibly the most perfect food made by nature.1235678900000000poiuytrewqasdfghjkmnbvcxzdwfcegvhbtjyuki8lokjhgf dsaasdfghjkhgfdsasdfghjkhgfrewqwertyhjuyhtrewq

Eggs contain high quality protein, healthy fats and antioxidants. The high quality fats are found in the yolks, so enough with the egg white omelets already. These oval shaped miracles are abundant in choline, of which 90 percent of the population has a deficiency. Choline helps with memory, lethargy and brain fog. Can you say the same for sugary cereals, evil lobbyists?

To this day there are people alerting the village elders to stay away from eggs because of their high cholesterol content. As we learned in *My Big Fat Life Transformation*, eating dietary fat does not directly add fat to your waistline. The same concept holds true here: eating foods high in cholesterol does not raise your bad cholesterol. In fact, those processed sugary cereals are the real culprit contributing to the LDL cholesterol floating around, waiting for the right moment to send you into cardiac arrest.

Check out stories of people who live past 100 years. Most of them proudly proclaim to eat eggs every day. If they were the tiny nuggets of death most lobbyists claim them to be, why are people who eat eggs daily living past 115 years?

Now that I convinced you to eat all the eggs, please know egg labels can get confusing. They even confuse me, and I've been doing this for a while. Even though you may not be able to find the highest quality eggs listed in your area, do your best. This is what you want to look for:

- Free range or pastured organic eggs for higher nutrient quality
- Cage free is different than free range - chickens need access to outdoors (you want free range)
- Organic means they were fed organic feed, so they are not storing pesticides. Not adding pesticides to your already toxic body is a plus!
- Try to buy locally raised eggs if you can.

Even with all of this egg knowledge tucked away in my brain, some days eggs still are not my favorite. Melting cheese over eggs makes them delicious, but my body does not always process cheese well so I avoid it when I can. I like to save my cheese binges up for delicious recipes like sausage crust pizza or cheesy Buffalo ranch chicken and cauliflower rice.

Most people I know make boring eggs. That is probably the reason I did not like them growing up. They tasted so eggy. Boring no more! I provide three spectacular and easy egg recipes in this cookbook. Feel free to eat them for breakfast, lunch or dinner. These recipes are the only eggs I can personally eat every day.

The recipes contain heavy cream. If you are like me and do not process dairy well, feel free to substitute coconut milk. Aim for the highest fat, lowest carb coconut milk you can find. As with any of the recipes in this book, if a recipe contains an ingredient you are not fond of or you are deathly allergic to, take it out. Like eggs. If you have an egg allergy that will send you into anaphylactic shock, don't make bruschetta BBQ scrambled eggs because I included the recipe in this cookbook. Most people assume that part is obvious. Trust me, not always as obvious as I thought.

There is another tidbit I discovered about eggs that you probably will not read in any other cookbook out there. We have separate plates and mixing bowls for our eggs. These dishes do not go into the dishwasher ever. For a long time we noticed out glass dishes had a funky smell to them, especially the water glasses. We went so far as to get a new dishwasher because the smell was awful. Who wants fresh water from a foul smelling glass?

It turns out the dishwasher was just fine. There is something about raw and runny eggs that gives plates a funky smell. When these dishes are washed with other glass dishes in a dishwasher, the smell can spread. This odd tidbit may have just saved someone five hundred dollars on the purchase of a new dishwasher.

Easy Scrambled Eggs

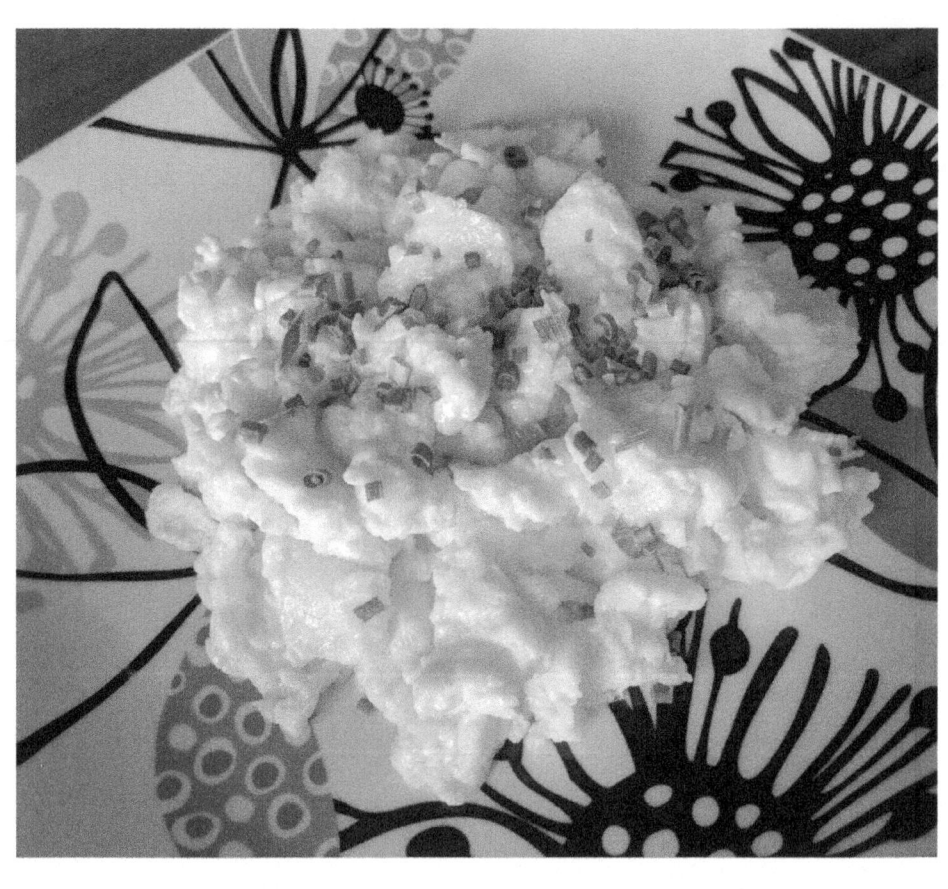

Ingredients:

- 4 large eggs
- 1 tablespoon butter
- ½ teaspoon minced garlic
- 2 tablespoons heavy whipping cream
- Chives, black pepper and sea salt to season

Directions:

- Melt butter in skillet over low heat.
- Once melted, add minced garlic. Cook until lightly browned, or 2-3 minutes.
- Whisk eggs in mixing bowl with heavy cream.
- Add egg mixture to skillet.
- Cook over medium heat, scrambling occasionally.
- Garnish with chives, salt and pepper to taste.

*Makes 2 servings

Tip: I like to pour creamy garlic pesto sauce over eggs for tasty, high-fat variety.

Garlic & Herb Scrambled Eggs

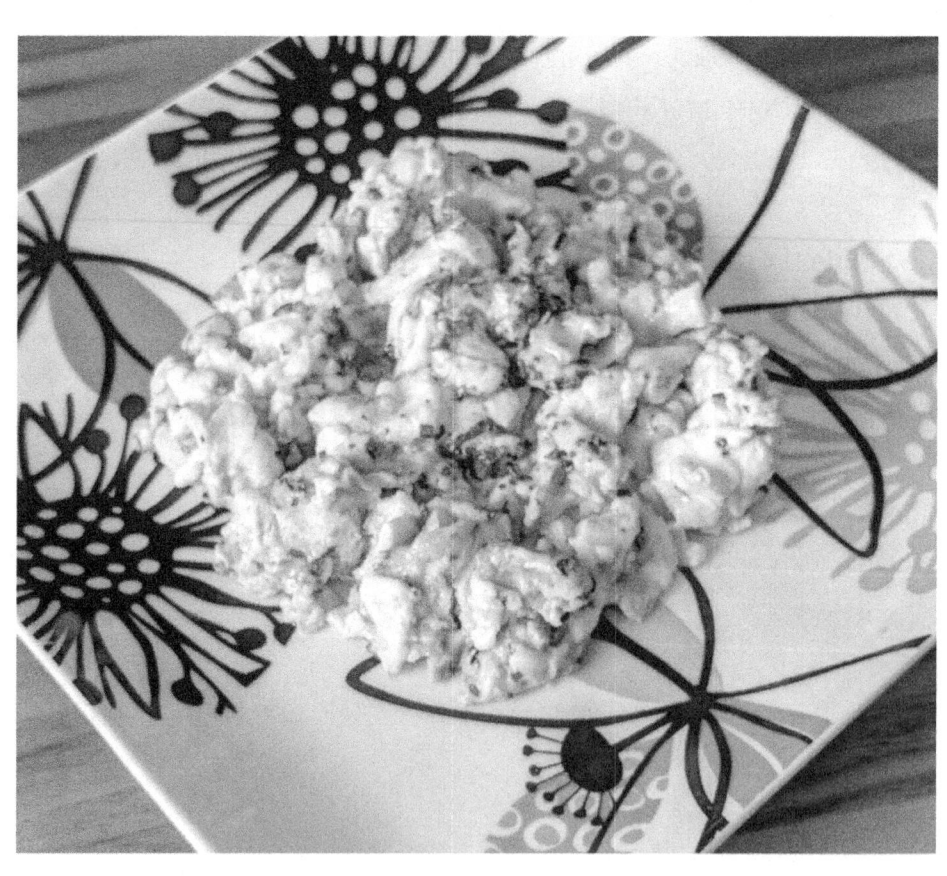

Ingredients:

- 4 large eggs
- 1 tablespoon garlic herb butter
- 2 tablespoons heavy whipping cream

Directions:

- Melt garlic herb butter in skillet over low heat.
- Whisk eggs in mixing bowl with heavy cream.
- Once butter melts, add egg mixture to skillet.
- Cook over medium heat, scrambling occasionally.
- Garnish with extra garlic herb butter.

*Makes 2 servings

BBQ & Bruschetta Scrambled Eggs

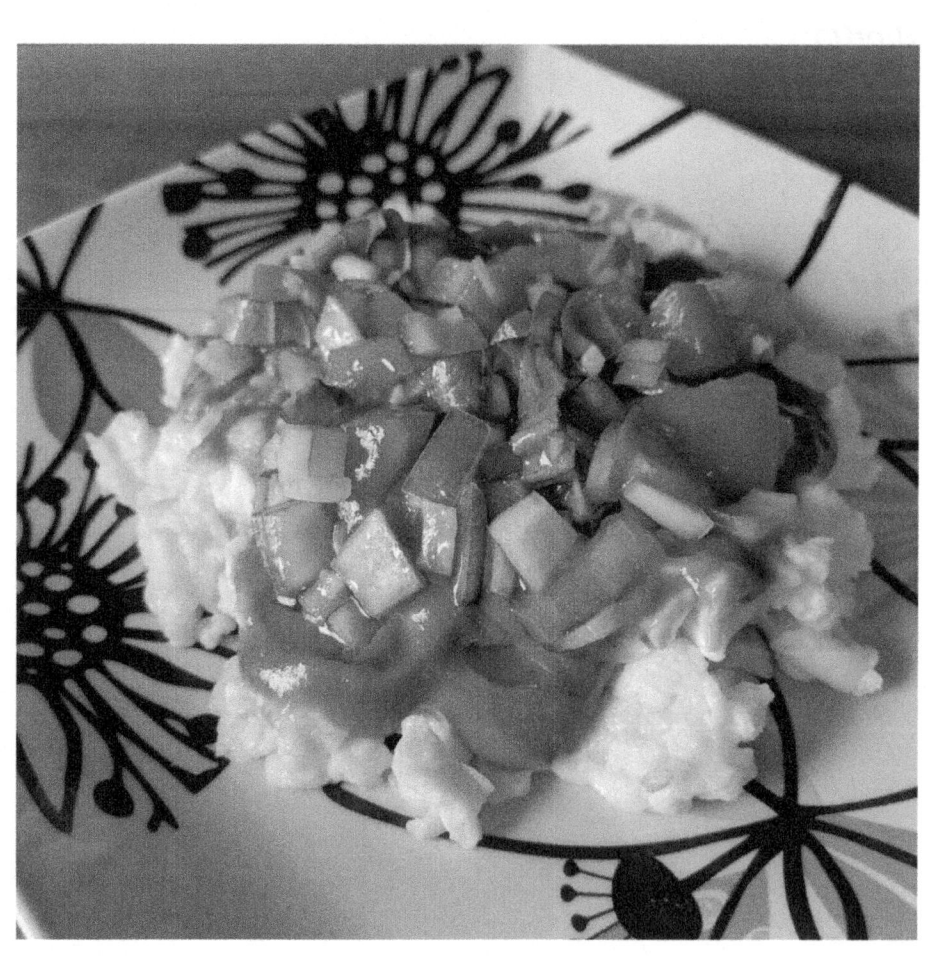

Ingredients:

- 4 large eggs
- 1 tablespoon butter
- ½ teaspoon minced garlic
- 2 tablespoons heavy whipping cream
- 4 tablespoons low sugar BBQ sauce
- 4 tablespoons bruschetta

Directions:

- Melt butter in skillet over low heat.
- Once butter melts, add minced garlic to skillet. Cook until lightly browned, or 2-3 minutes.
- Whisk eggs and heavy cream in mixing bowl.
- Add egg mixture to skillet.
- Cook over medium heat, scrambling occasionally.
- Plate and garnish with BBQ sauce and bruschetta.

*Recipe makes 2 servings

Lazy Gourmet

Grab and Go

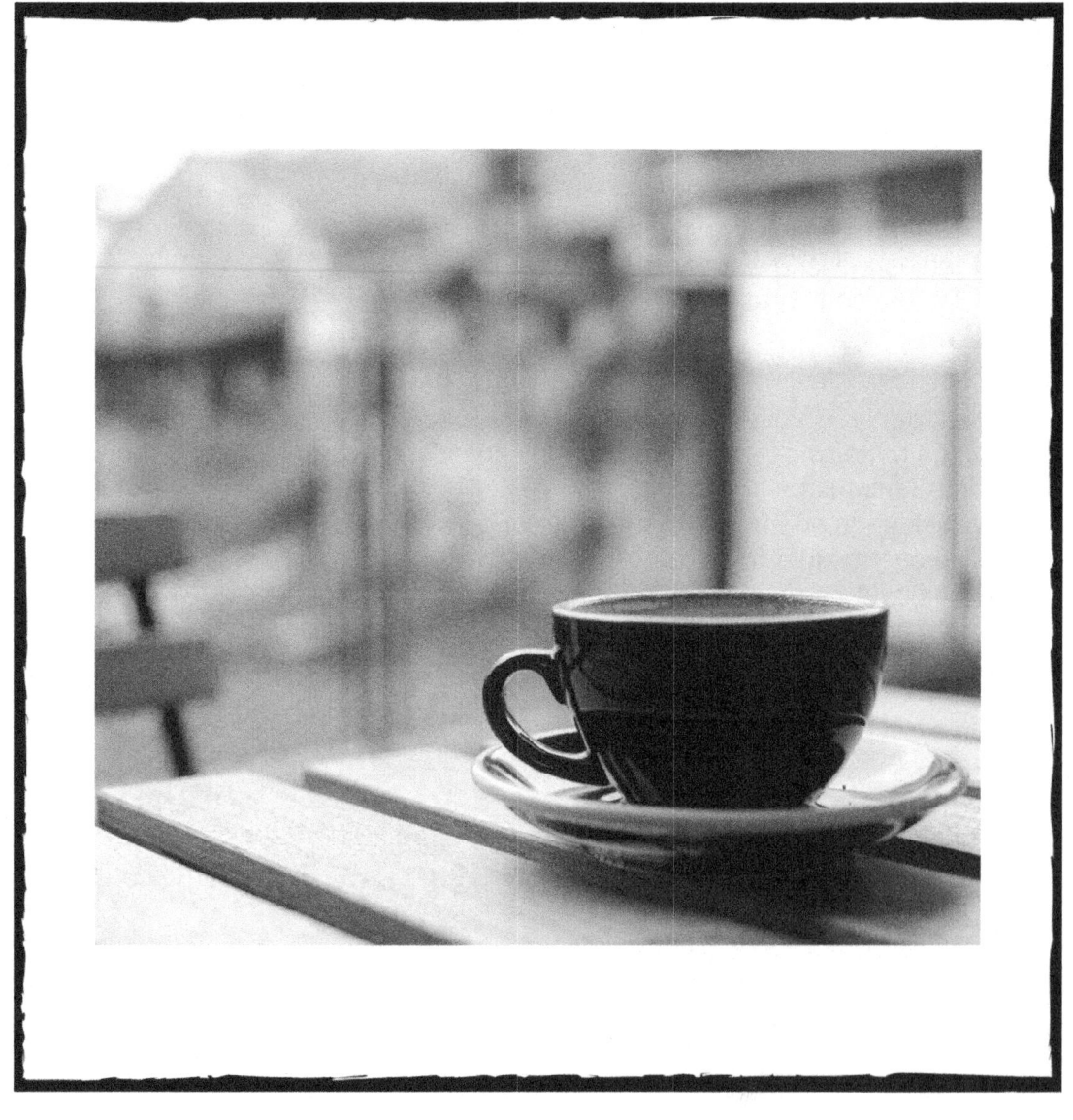

Grab and Go: Low-Carb

The remaining breakfasts listed in this cookbook are not typical of most low-carb, high-fat diets as far as breakfasts are concerned. Unfortunately their sugary counterparts *are* typical of the standard American diet, aptly coined the SAD diet.

The good news is the crumbly PB bars, dark chocolate protein cupcakes and chocolate pecan balls are not filled with sugar the way most breakfast grab and go items like poptarts or donuts are. Score!

When I am not fasting for breakfast and I do not have time to cook eggs, I grab a few of these treats to take to go. They are delicious and filled with healthy fats. I also like to eat one or two of these items at home following a keto cold buster tea with Perfect Keto Unflavored Collagen added in. This makes an easy gut healing breakfast that also keeps me satiated.

I recently changed my collagen from Great Lakes Collagen in the green can to Perfect Keto Unflavored Collagen. I still believe Great Lakes makes an awesome product, but for those of us following a ketogenic diet, consuming a dose of collagen without fat to slow the absorption down can result in gluconeogenesis. If you do not know what that means, it is a process that can kick some people out of ketosis. Adding fat in with your dose of collagen can slow the absorption rate, which will keep you in ketosis.

Perfect Keto Unflavored Collagen has MCT oil added to their product for this very reason. I even coyly slip this product into my children's low-sugar juice to get them the healthy protein and fats their growing bodies and brains require. This blend mixes much more easily than the Great Lakes collagen as well, so they remain unaware of the healthy juice I am slipping them.

If you are in the market for Perfect Keto Unflavored Collagen, please click on my link on my website as I am an affiliate for their products. This means I get paid a small commision when someone uses my link. I will only become an affiliate for products I know, love and trust. This makes Perfect Keto a product I personally know, love and trust for my family.

Speaking of perfect, before we start this section is the perfect time to point out **I no longer use any artificial sweeteners in my recipes**. This includes the more "natural" artificial sweeteners like stevia or Swerve. If you are accustomed to highly sweetened food like the rest of the world, some of these recipes may be too bitter for your palate that has been highly trained with extra sweetness because sweeteners are added to practically every food on the planet. If you have not weaned yourself off of artificial sweeteners yet, nor do you have plans to in the future, you may want to add your sweetener of choice to the remaining breakfast recipes and drinks. Ditto for the fat bomb section of this cookbook.

Dark Chocolate Protein Cupcakes

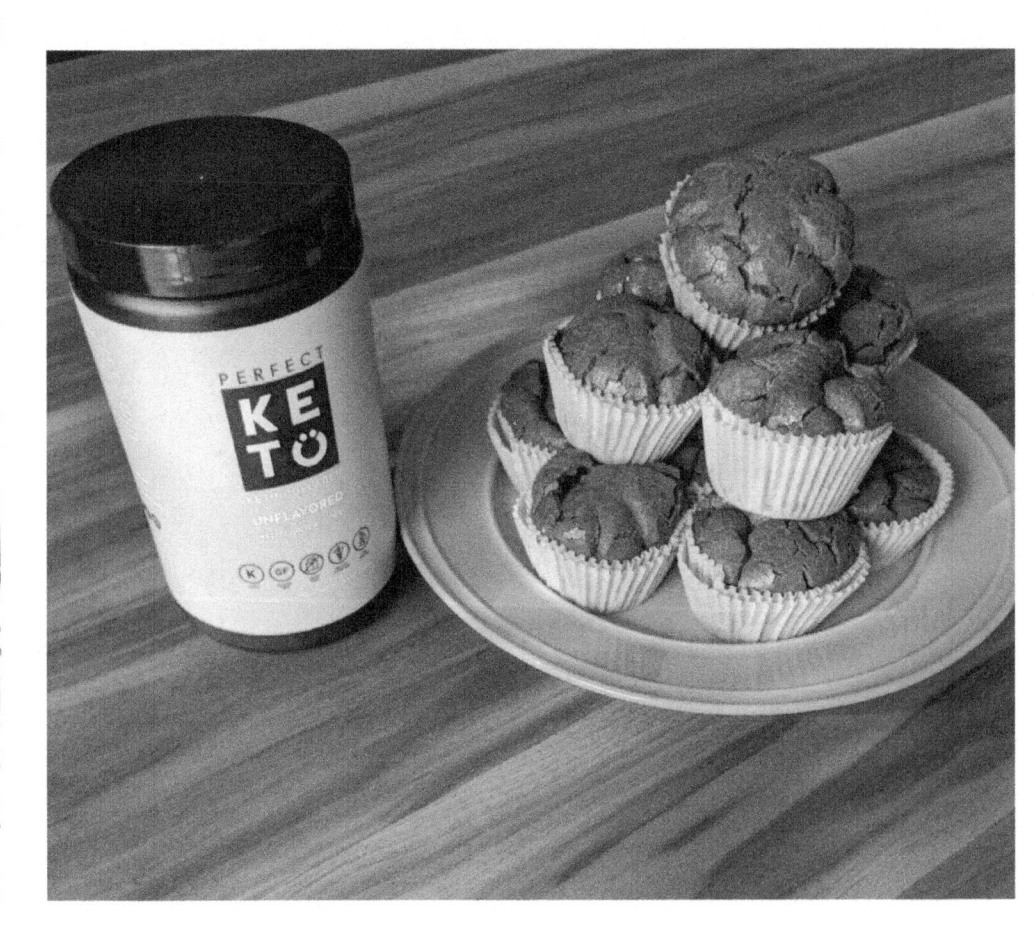

Ingredients:

- 7 ounces dark chocolate
- 8 tablespoons butter
- 1 teaspoon vanilla extract
- 4 large eggs
- 4 tablespoons heavy whipping cream
- 3 ounces Perfect Keto Unflavored Collagen

Directions:

- Preheat oven to 350 degrees.
- Layer cupcake tins with liners.
- Melt dark chocolate and butter together over low heat.
- Once melted, set aside to cool.
- In a separate bowl, combine eggs, heavy cream and collagen together with hand mixer.
- Pour vanilla extract into chocolate mixture and stir.
- Slowly combine egg, heavy cream and collagen mixture with chocolate mixture. Stir with whisk or hand mixer on low as you combine.
- Pour into cupcake tins.
- Bake for 25 minutes, or until set in center.

*Recipe makes 12 cupcakes

Crumbly PB Bars

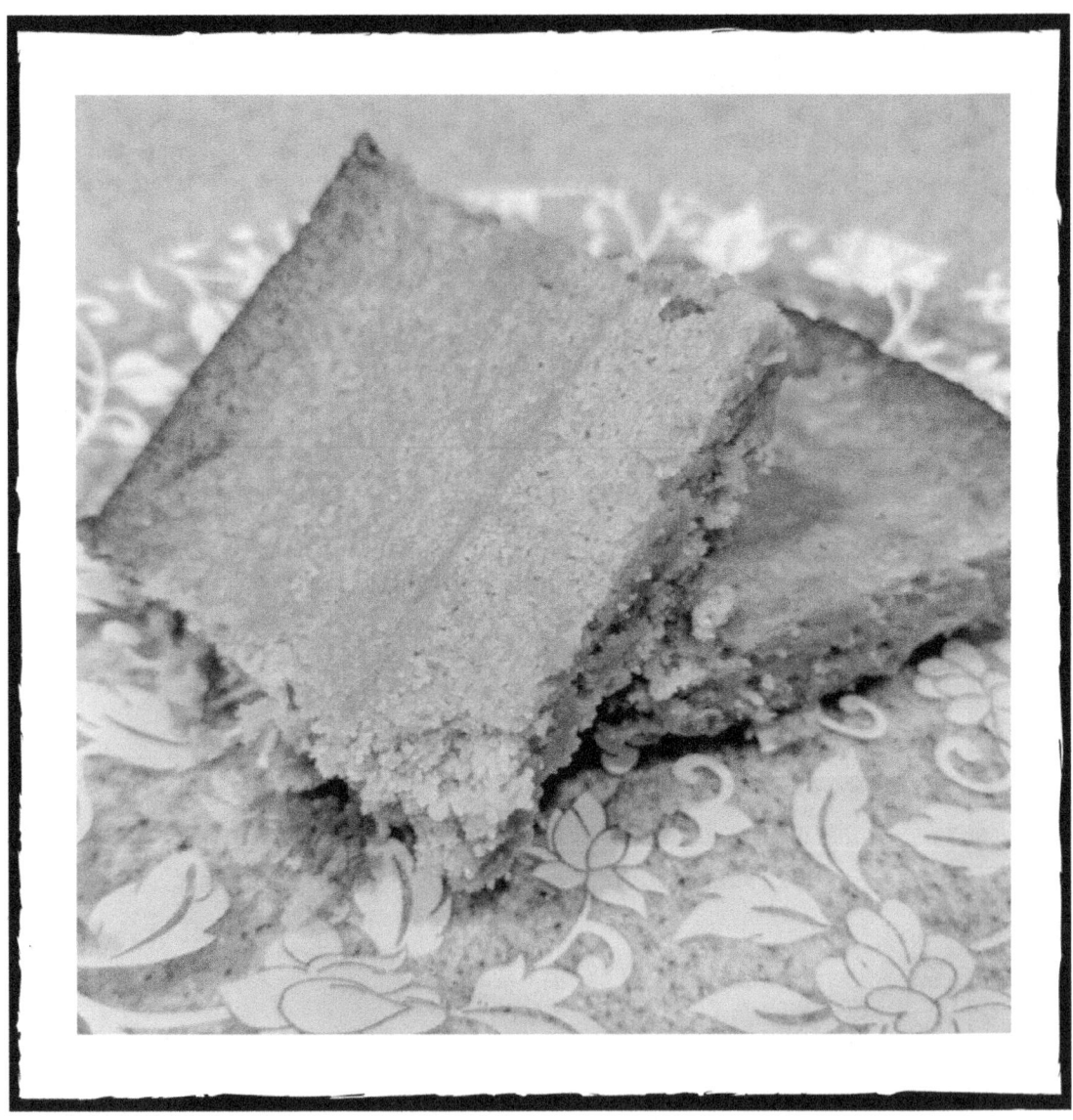

Ingredients:

- 1 cup peanut butter
- 12 tablespoons butter, softened
- 4 tablespoons coconut oil
- 1 large egg
- ¼ cup coconut flour
- 1 tablespoon collagen
- 1 teaspoon baking powder
- 1 teaspoon vanilla extract
- Nonstick cooking spray

Directions:

- Preheat oven to 350 degrees.
- Add peanut butter, butter, coconut oil, baking powder, collagen and vanilla extract to a mixing bowl. Combine ingredients with a hand mixer.
- Once combined, add egg and mix again.
- Add in coconut flour and mix ingredients. Do not over mix once coconut flour has been added.
- Pour mixture into 9×9 greased baking tin. Flatten with spatula.
- Bake approximately 30 minutes, or until outside is slightly brown and inside is cooked.
- Allow to cool before serving.

*Recipe makes 16 bars

*TIP: Bars may be crumbly on the first day. They harden overnight, but will still crumble slightly.

Chocolate Pecan Balls

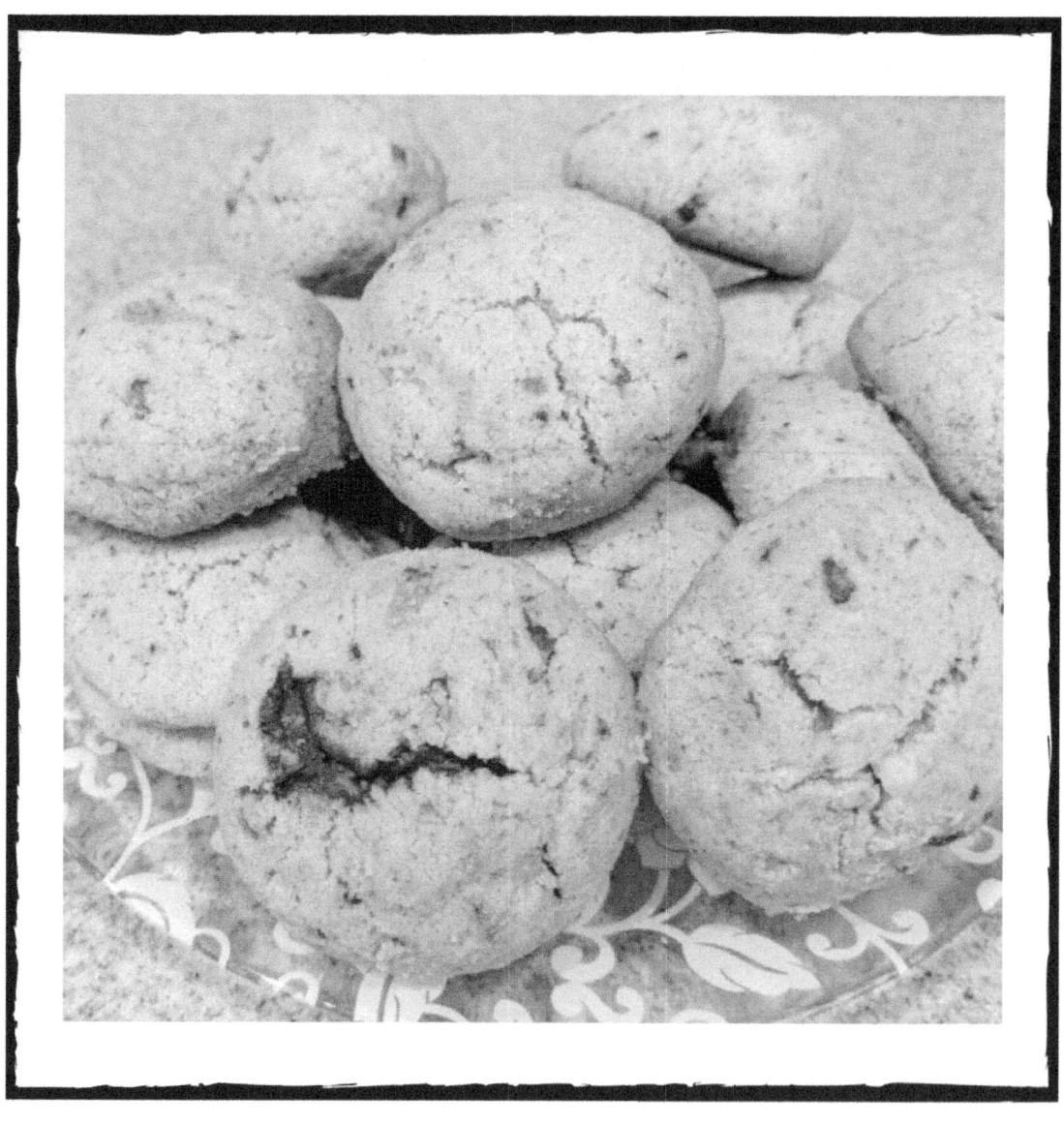

Ingredients:

- 8 tablespoons butter, softened
- 4 tablespoons coconut oil
- 1 & ½ cups almond flour
- ½ cup almond butter
- 1 teaspoon vanilla extract
- 1 & ½ teaspoons baking powder
- 1 tablespoon collagen
- 1 large egg
- 2 ounces dark chocolate, chopped
- ⅓ cup pecans, chopped
- Nonstick cooking spray

Directions:

- Preheat oven to 350 degrees.
- With hand mixer, combine butter, coconut oil, almond butter, vanilla extract, baking powder and collagen.
- Once combined, add egg and mix again.
- Add almond flour and mix until combined. Do not over mix flour, as this may cause recipe to dry out.
- Add in chopped chocolate and pecans. Mix with hands.
- Form into 1.5 inch balls and place onto greased cookie sheet.
- Bake 20 – 25 minutes, or until bottoms are golden and center is cooked.

Lazy Gourmet Drinks

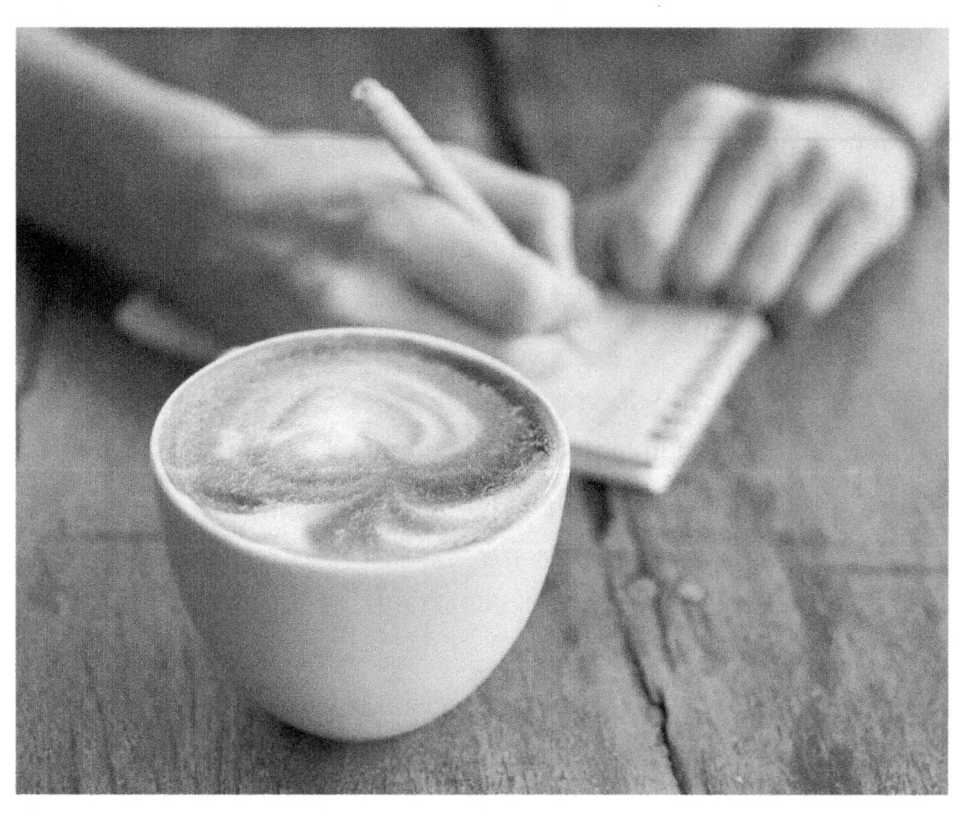

Breakfast Drinks

If you are among the poor digestion folks I talked about above, you may want to try out some of the hot chocolate recipes for breakfast in place of food you have to chew. Mixing in collagen is a great way to get nutrients where they are needed most. If you want to learn more about the reason I add collagen to so many recipes, read here.

If you have poor digestion, drinking meals is an easy way to get nutrients you may not receive otherwise. The nutrients are already broken down, which means less work for your overworked body. Keep in mind most people will feel fuller longer when they actually chew their food. Feel free to drink your breakfast until you have better digestion. Once you fix that up, you can go back to chewing food like a normal human.

If digesting fats well isn't your thing, be careful with how much fat you add to your breakfast drinks. If it has been some time since you and healthy fats have been friends and then you decide to drink a lot of heavy cream all at once, stay close to a bathroom that day. Maybe add less fat tomorrow and every day after until you take the steps to correct this. When I exclaim, "Eat fat, get healthy!" I do not include singing "diarrhea, diarrhea, cha cha cha," all day, everyday.

This is also the part where you can get fat by eating too much fat. If you cannot digest the fat you eat, you will feel miserable, you will store some of that fat as toxins (extra body fat) and you will have a spitfire rage shooting out of your backside most of the time. Not fun. Not healthy.

Some of the symptoms of not digesting fat well include bloating in your lower abdomen, diarrhea, acne, light colored stool, nausea (especially when you add more fat), itchiness, gas and if you had your gallbladder removed but did not add an ox bile supplement. If you are experiencing these symptoms while partaking in a low-carb, high-fat diet, you need to ease into the high-fat part more slowly. You also need to take the digestion course so you can learn the steps to improve these symptoms. This will make your life easier. Not having a spitfire rage shooting out of your backside will make life easier. You might have to trust me on that part if that's not your current norm.

Speaking of improving problems, I also listed the keto cold buster tea under the breakfast section. This is one of my favorite drinks to start my day. When you add collagen to the tea on an empty stomach, this is one of the best ways to begin to heal your gut lining. Healing your gut lining has So. Many. Health. Benefits. Too many to get into in this cookbook, but check in with my website eatingfatisthenewskinny.com every now and then for updated blogs on this topic.

The keto cold buster tea is also helpful when you feel a cold coming on, hence the creative name. When some people begin a low-carb, high-fat diet, their pH levels can be affected adversely. The apple cider vinegar and lemon juice can help balance pH levels. I try to drink this with added collagen in the morning, but I will drink just the tea a few more times each day if I feel a cold approaching. This drink typically knocks the cold out before it has a chance to get going. That's a drastic change from my yo-yoing past where I had sinus infections for at least half of the year.

The tea has other benefits like aiding in proper digestion of food. ACV can add acid if you are lacking stomach acid, but not enough where you require additional HCL supplementation. I added sea salt to the drink in the case of those who need to find a way to get more electrolytes. Feel free to leave the salt out if your electrolytes feel balanced.

Creamy Keto Hot Chocolate

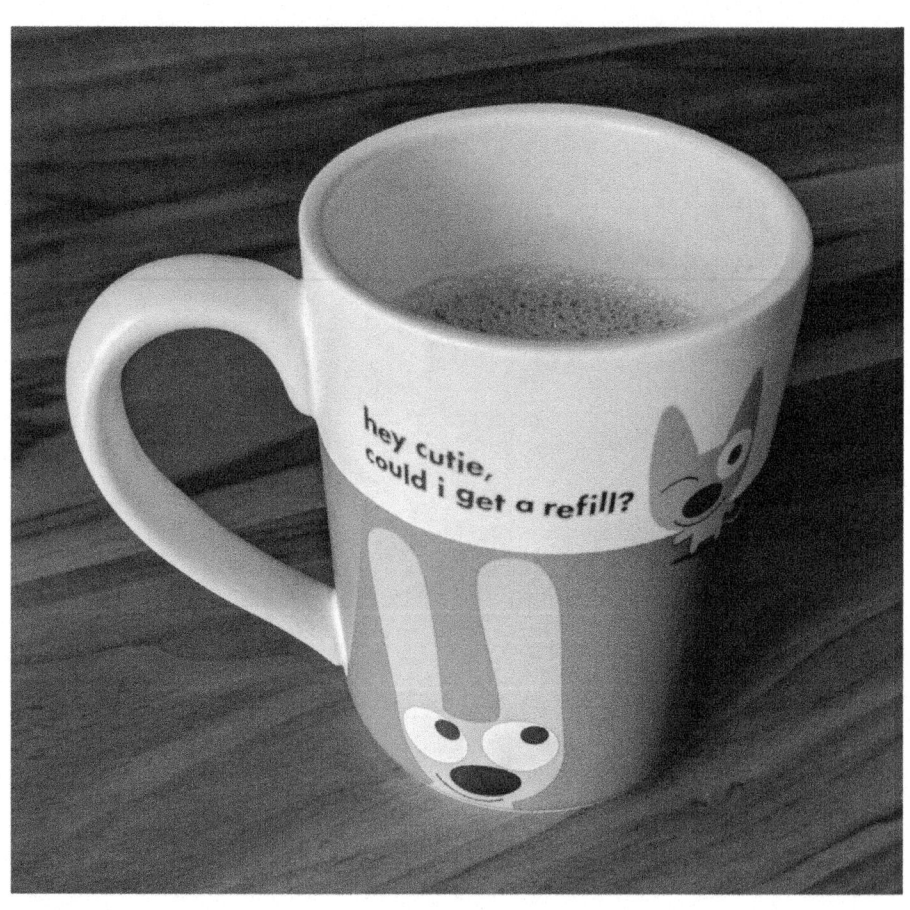

Ingredients:

- 4 ounces water
- 4 ounces heavy whipping cream
- ½ ounce dark chocolate
- ½ ounce collagen

Directions:

- Warm cream and water in small saucepan on stove over medium heat until hot but not boiling, or approximately 5 minutes.
- Once warmed, remove from heat. Stir in collagen and chocolate. Continue to stir until chocolate is melted.
- For an extra frothy hot chocolate, pour into an immersion blender. Blend on high for 30 seconds.

TIPS: Adjust heavy cream / water ratio for desired fat & creaminess. If substituting coconut milk, do not combine with water; use a full 8 ounces of coconut milk.

Salted Caramel
Hot Chocolate

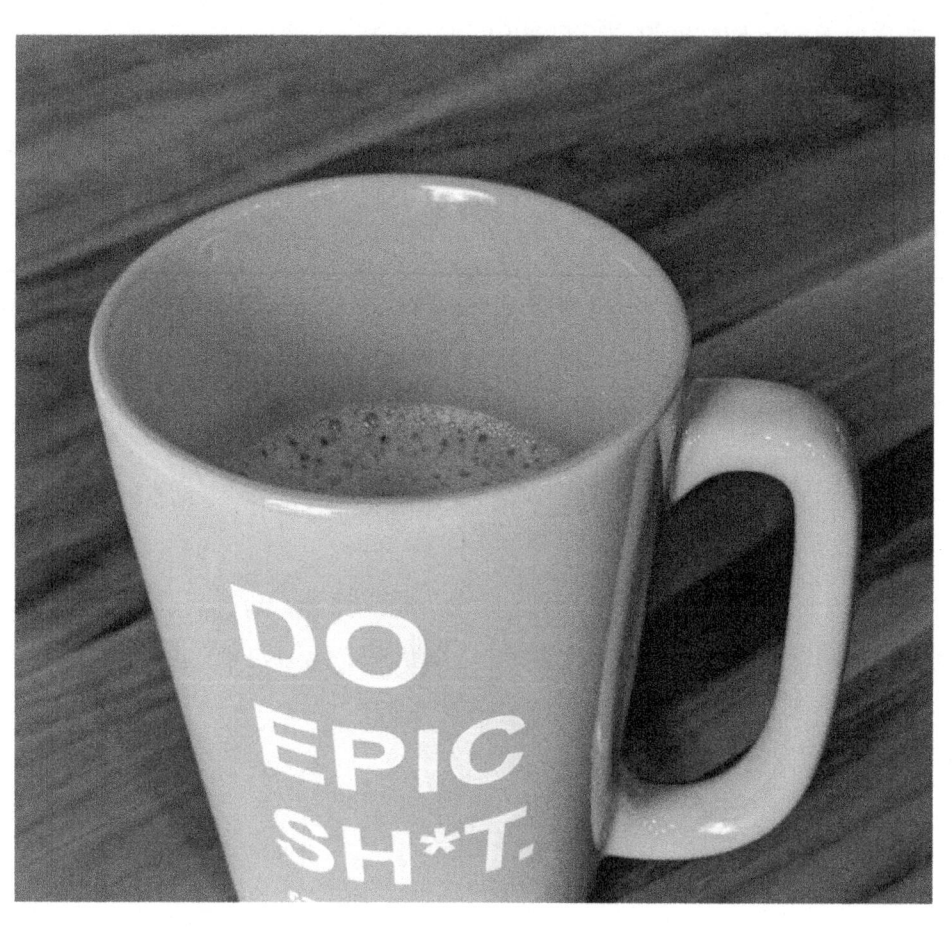

Ingredients:

- 4 ounces water
- 3 ounces heavy whipping cream
- 1 tablespoon butter
- ½ ounce dark chocolate
- ½ ounce collagen
- Pinch of salt

Directions:

- Warm cream, butter and water in small saucepan on stove over medium heat until hot but not boiling, or approximately 5 minutes.
- Once warmed, remove from heat. Stir in collagen and chocolate.
- Stir until chocolate is melted. Add pinch of salt.
- For an extra frothy hot chocolate, pour into an immersion blender. Blend on high for 30 seconds.

*TIPS: Adjust heavy cream / water ratio for desired fat & creaminess. If substituting coconut milk, do not combine with water; use a full 8 ounces of coconut milk.

Keto Cold Buster Tea

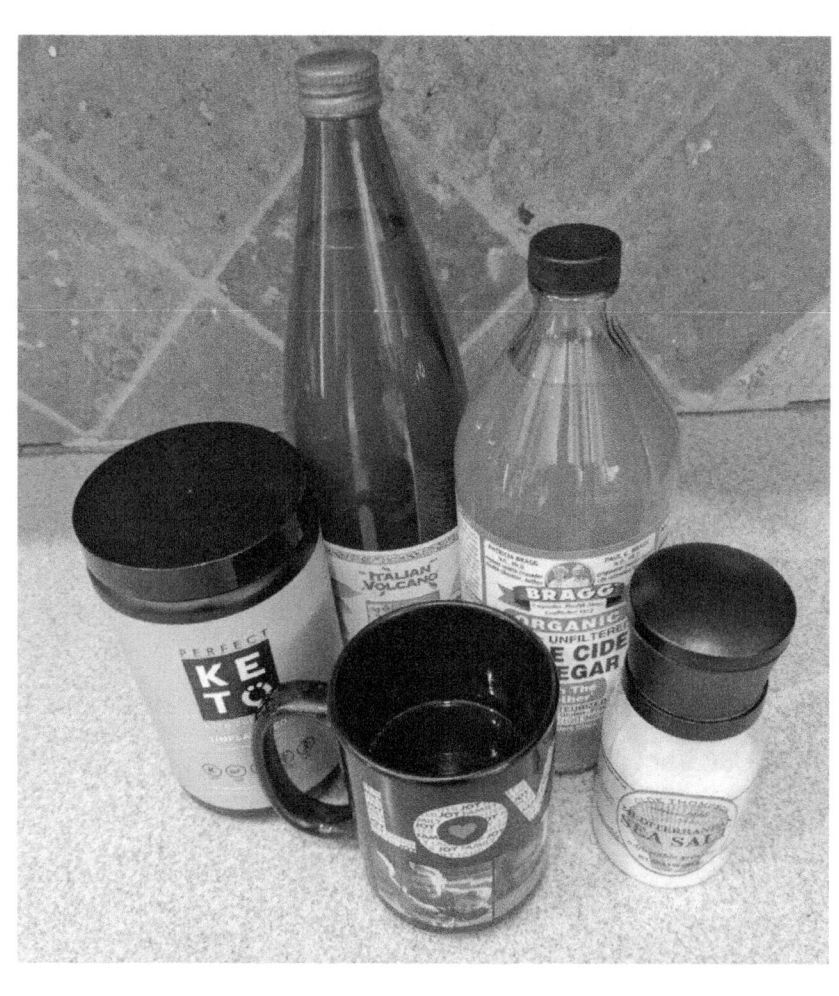

Ingredients:

- 8 ounces hot water
- 1 tablespoon apple cider vinegar
- 1 tablespoon lemon juice
- ½ teaspoon sea salt (only add for extra electrolytes)

Directions:

- Stir ingredients together and sip.

TIP: Stir in ½ ounce collagen for better gut health. Drink prior to your first meal of the day for maximum healing benefit.

Lazy Keto

Gourmet Meals

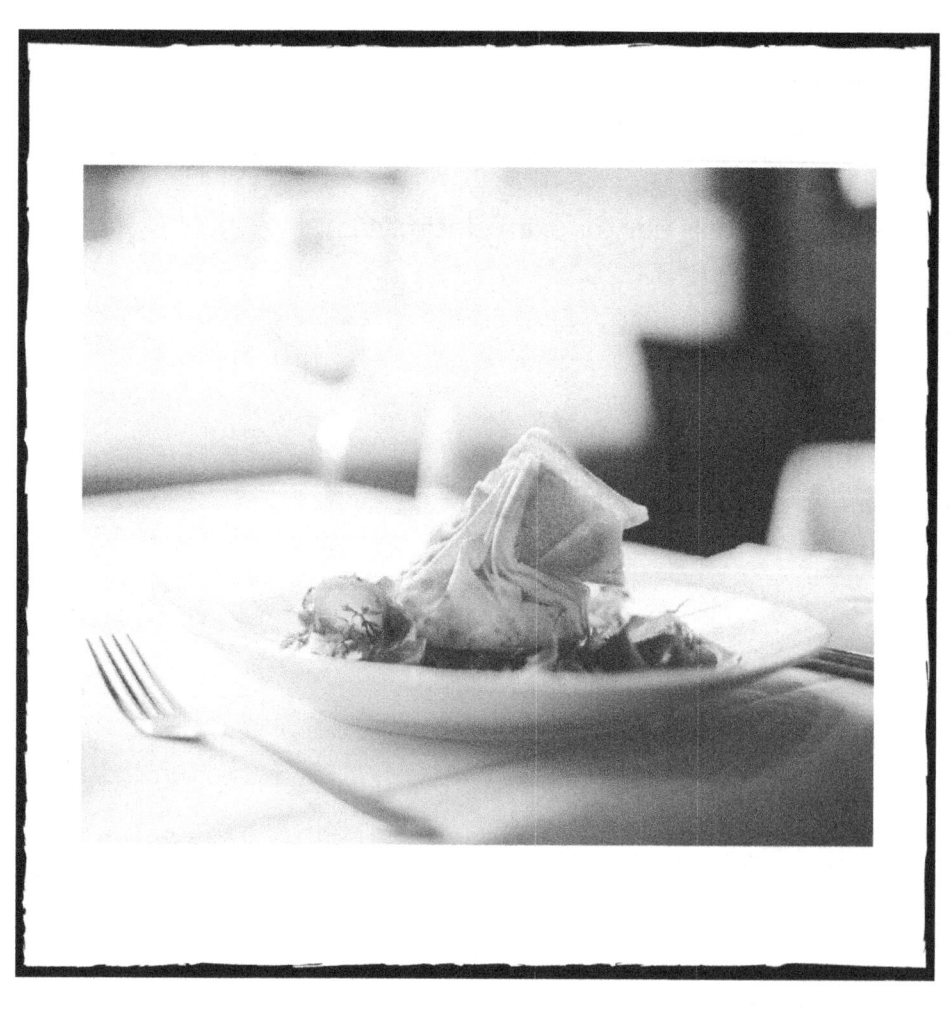

Lazy Keto Gourmet Meals

The Lazy Keto Gourmet meals in this cookbook are not only simple, but I would prefer many of these dishes over a night out at a fancy restaurant. I do not necessarily prefer the clean up aspect, but even that is sometimes a welcomed break from the chaos toddlers and a puppy bring to my day.

Being an overburdened mom of small kids, I do not have time to make complicated dinners. Most of the meals found in this cookbook have easy prep work and are simple to cook. The majority of the meals included take less than 30 minutes start to finish, and that time includes having to break up toddler fights as they run around the kitchen while I am cooking.

If you find meals you really love but somehow have even less time to cook than I do, make large batches and store them in the freezer to reheat later. You can even package them separately to reheat for lunch at work if you prefer a tasty home cooked meal that will make your co-workers drool.

You may also notice I am a little heavy handed on the garlic. I've always been a huge garlic fan since an early age. If any of the ingredients used are too much for your taste, feel free to use less. I use a lot of garlic for the taste factor, as well as the health benefits. I also obviously want to assure vampires stay far, far away.

Lazy Gourmet Chicken

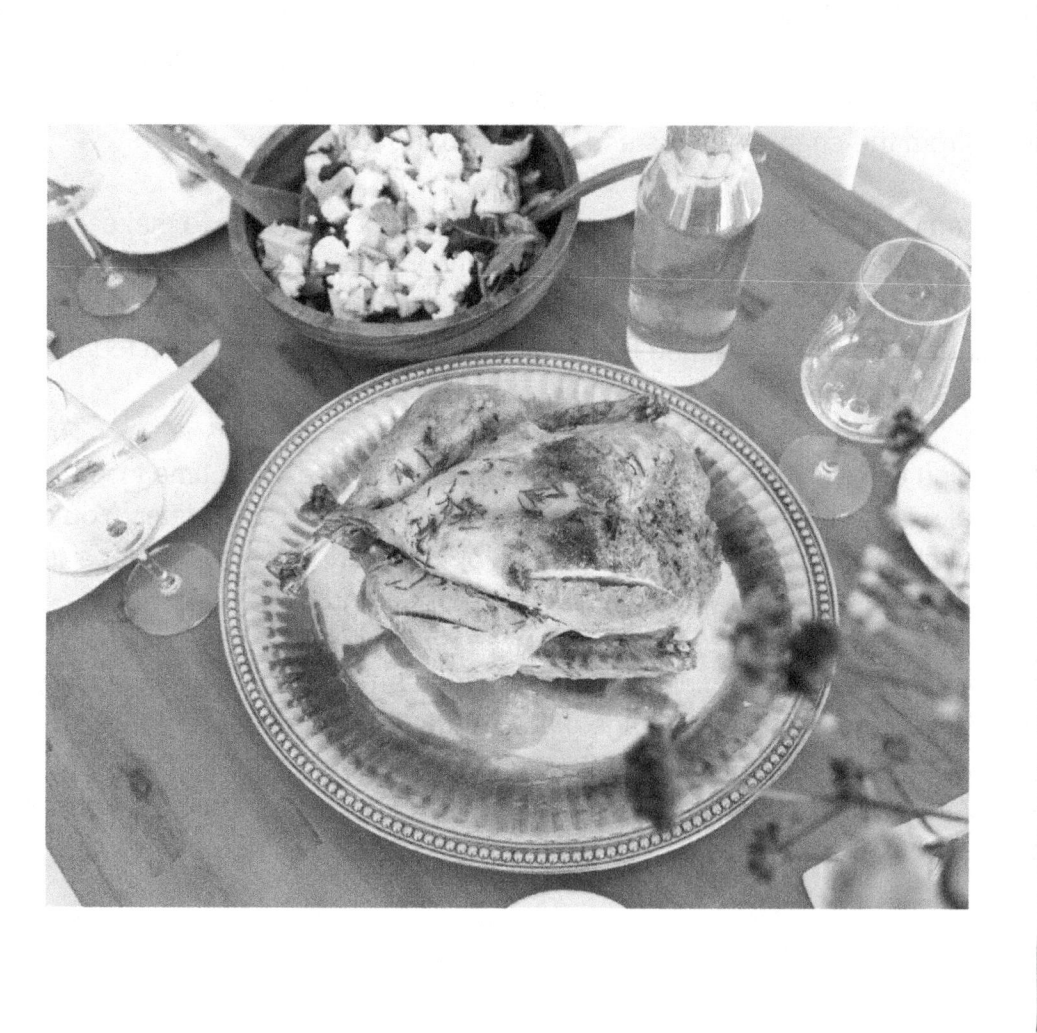

Lazy Gourmet Chicken

If you have been in the dieting world of Weight Watchers, SlimFast, Jenny Craig or the like for some time, your go to meal is going to be chicken. Boneless, skinless, tasteless chicken breasts to be more specific. I know you. I've been you. Chicken breasts have always been the go to healthy choice among fitness gurus everywhere. Chicken breasts are lean, low in calories and contain a lot of filling protein.

Chicken breasts are not always the best option for a low-carb, high-fat diet. If you like chicken thighs, choose that option. If you still prefer chicken breasts, be sure to add plenty of high-fat, delicious sauces to the chicken. Without the added fat, the high protein content and levels of arginine are enough to throw anyone out of ketosis. Every once in a while, as your digestion improves and your tastes change, give chicken thighs another chance. They are especially delicious in the crock-pot meals.

I bought a food thermometer to assess when my chicken is ready. Before I took this step, I tended to overcook chicken. This makes them rubbery and not very tasty. I cook chicken to an internal temperature of 165 degrees. Anything higher equates to rubber.

Mediterranean Chicken

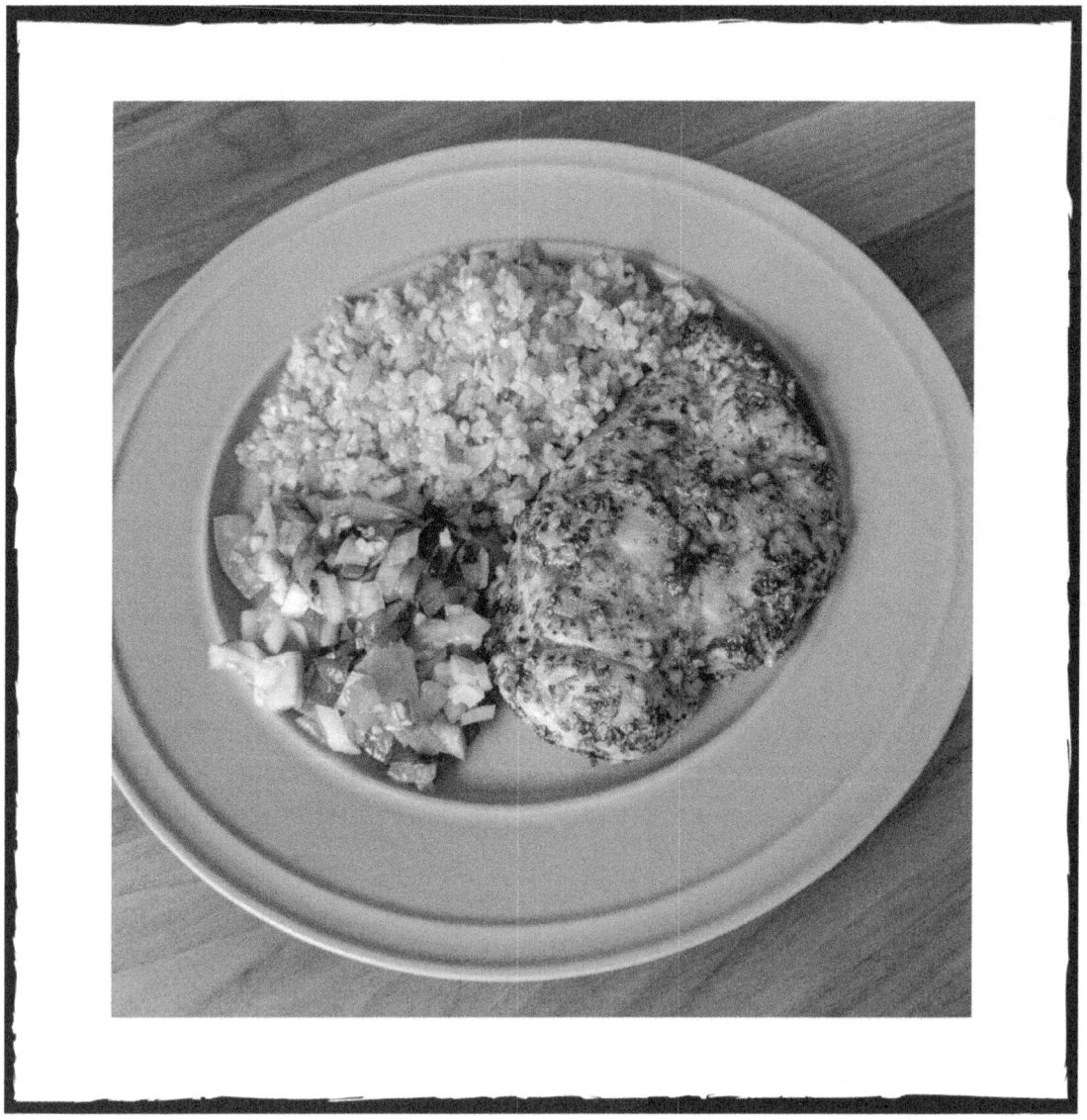

Ingredients:

- 1 pound chicken breasts or thighs
- 1/3 cup olive oil
- 1/4 cup coconut aminos
- 1/4 cup worcestershire sauce
- 2 teaspoons minced garlic
- 2 tablespoons basil
- 1 tablespoon oregano
- 1 teaspoon black pepper
- Nonstick cooking spray

Directions:

- Place all ingredients (except chicken) in a ziploc bag. Close and shake bag to mix marinade.
- Place chicken into ziploc bag and shake gently to coat chicken.
- Place chicken in fridge and allow to marinate for 30 minutes.
- Preheat oven to 350 degrees.
- Coat baking dish with nonstick cooking spray.
- Place marinated chicken into baking dish and bake for 25-30 minutes, or until chicken is cooked in center and juices run clear. If you have a food thermometer, check for an internal temperature of 165.

Garlic Butter Chicken

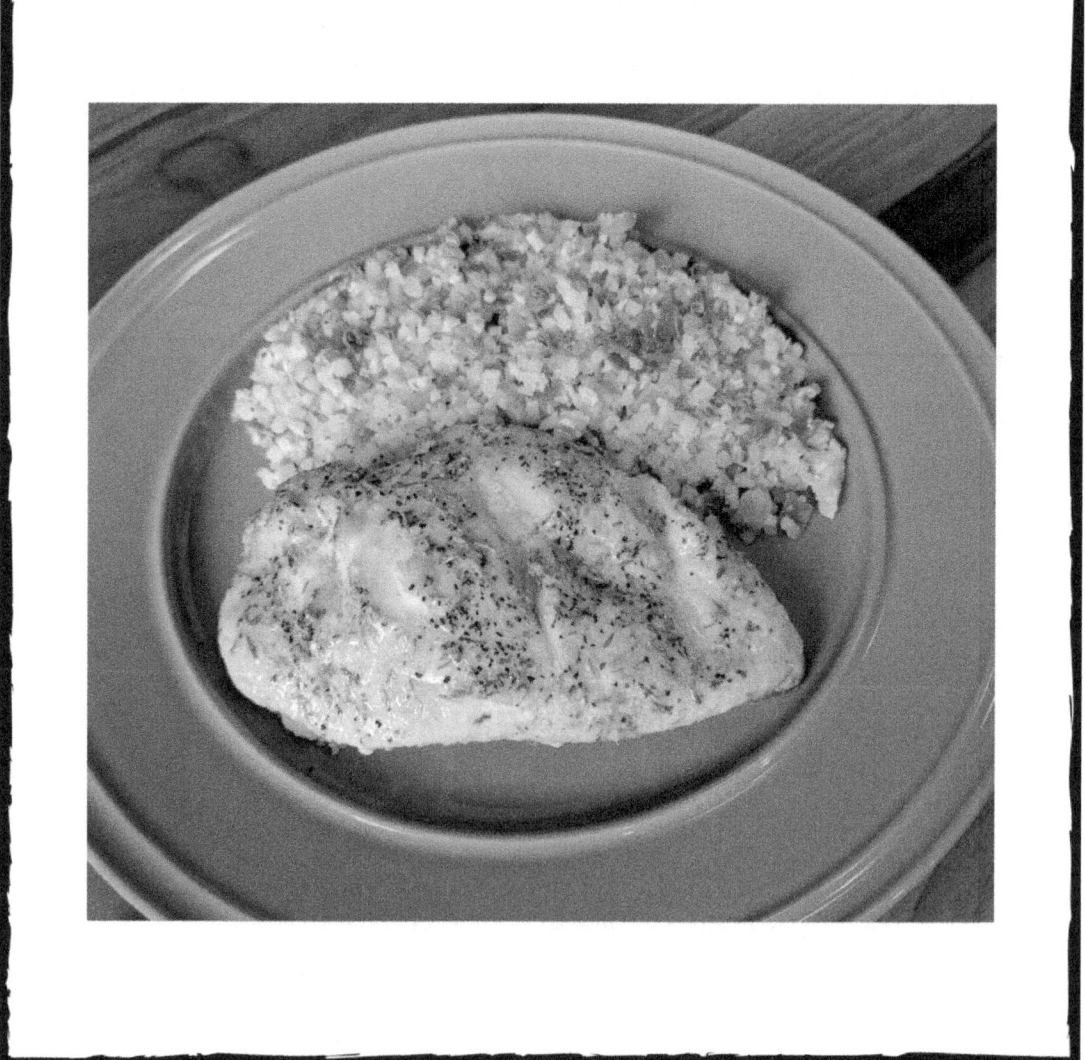

Ingredients:

- 2 large chicken breasts or thighs (approximately 1 pound)
- 3 tablespoons butter
- Garlic powder
- Thyme
- Sea salt
- Black pepper
- Nonstick cooking spray

Directions:

- Preheat oven to 350 degrees.
- Spray baking dish with nonstick cooking spray.
- Season chicken to taste with salt, pepper, garlic powder and thyme on both sides. Layer in baking dish.
- Make 3 slits per chicken breast or thigh. Cut close to bottom, but not all of the way through.
- Add one pat of butter (approximately ½ tablespoon) in between each slit.
- Bake for 25-30 minutes, or until chicken is cooked in center and juices run clear. If you have a food thermometer, check for an internal temperature of 165.
- Plate chicken and spoon melted butter on top of chicken.

Chicken Bacon Alfredo

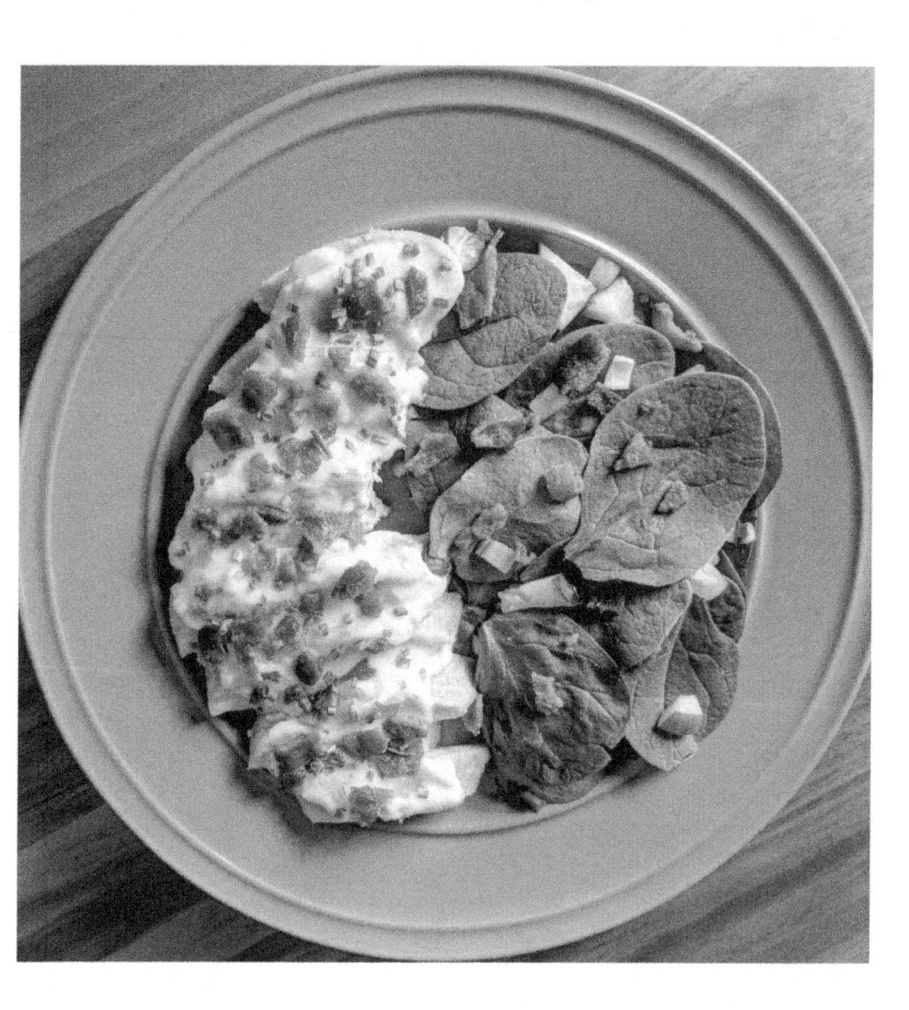

Ingredients:

- 1 pound chicken breasts or thighs
- 1 tablespoon butter
- ½ teaspoon minced garlic
- 1 cup heavy whipping cream
- ½ cup real bacon bits
- ¼ cup chopped green onions
- Sea salt
- Black pepper
- Garlic powder
- Nonstick cooking spray

Directions - Alfredo Sauce:

- Melt butter over low heat in saucepan.
- Add minced garlic to melted butter. Cook until lightly browned, or 2-3 minutes.
- Begin to add heavy cream to saucepan. Add ½ cup heavy cream to pan, stirring frequently. Once sauce thickens, repeat with additional ½ cup. Remove from heat once sauce thickens, typically 10-20 minutes.

Directions - Chicken Breasts or Thighs:

- Preheat oven to 350 degrees.
- Spray baking dish with nonstick cooking spray.
- Season both sides of chicken with salt, pepper and garlic.
- Bake for 25-30 minutes, or until chicken is cooked in center and juices run clear. If you have a food thermometer, check for an internal temperature of 165.

Combine:

- Slice chicken and top with a generous portion of sauce. Garnish with crispy bacon bits and green onions.

Buffalo Butter Chicken

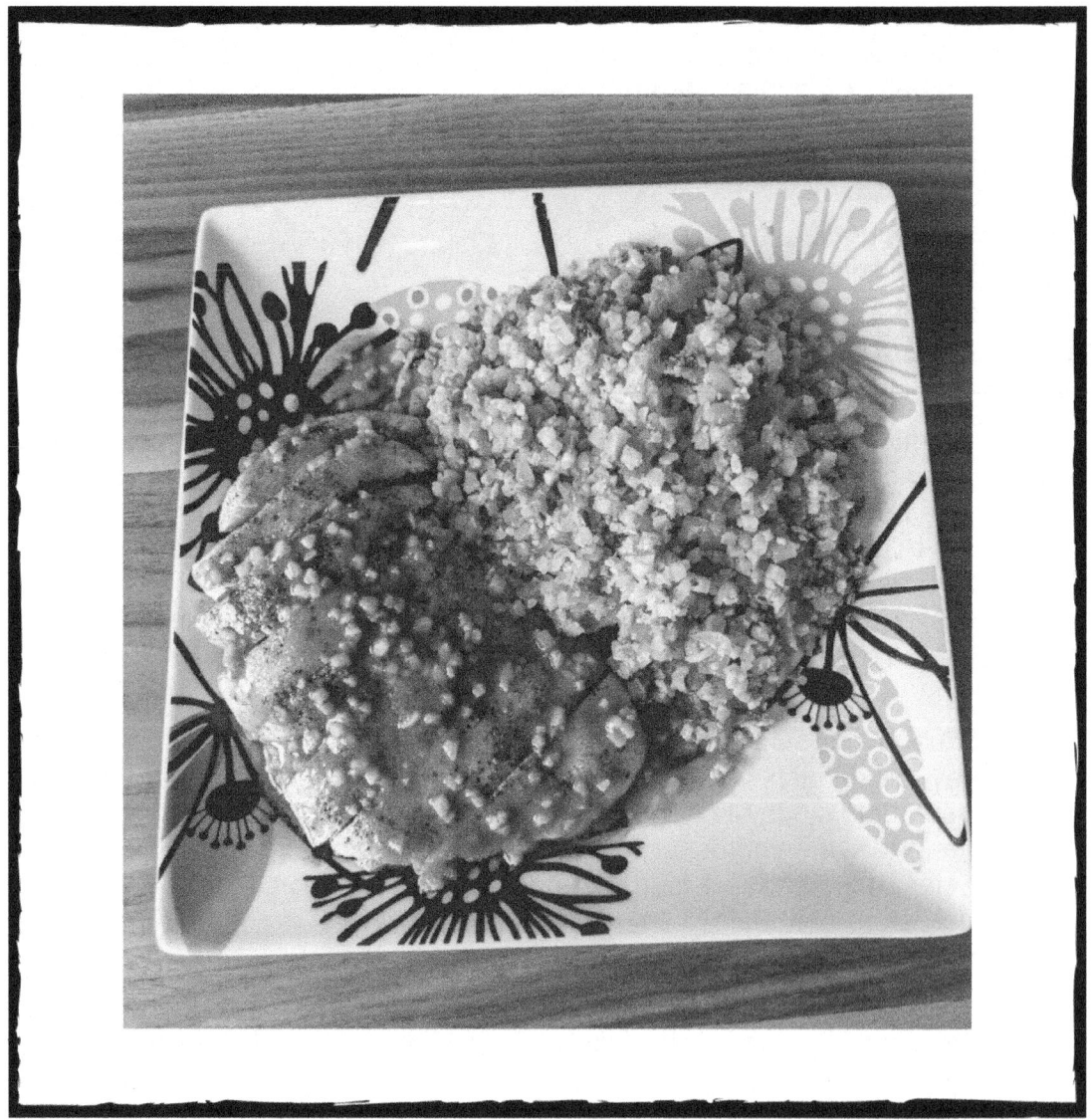

Ingredients:

- 1 pound chicken breasts or thighs
- Garlic powder, black pepper and sea salt to season chicken
- 4 tablespoons butter
- 2 teaspoons minced garlic
- ¼ cup Buffalo wing sauce
- ¼ teaspoon smoked paprika (or regular paprika)
- ¼ teaspoon cayenne pepper (optional for extra spicy)
- ¼ teaspoon sea salt
- Black pepper
- Nonstick cooking spray

Directions:

- Preheat oven to 350 degrees.
- Spray baking dish with nonstick cooking spray.
- Season both sides of chicken with garlic powder, black pepper and salt.
- Bake for 25-30 minutes, or until chicken is cooked in center and juices run clear. If you have a food thermometer, check for an internal temperature of 165.

While Chicken is Baking:

- In small saucepan, melt butter and minced garlic together on low.
- Once butter is melted, add Buffalo sauce, smoked paprika, cayenne pepper, sea salt and pepper. Stir well.
- Remove chicken from oven, slice and pour a generous amount of Buffalo butter sauce on top.

Cheesy Buffalo Ranch Chicken & Caulirice

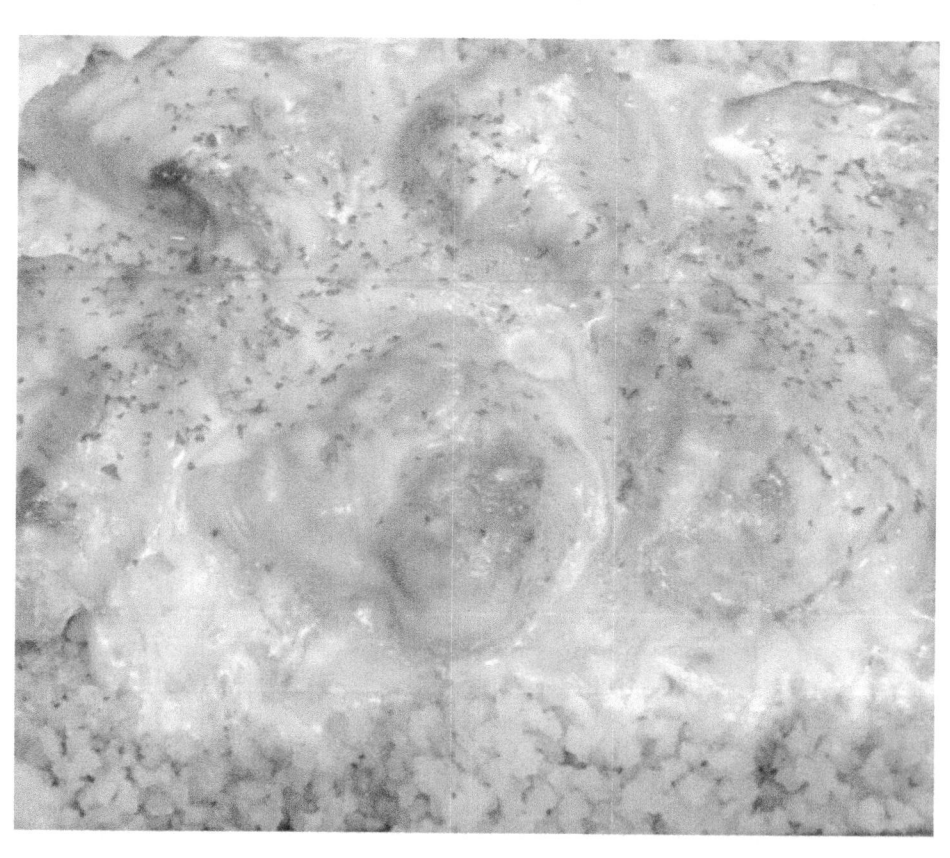

Ingredients:

- 1 pound boneless chicken breasts or thighs
- 6 ounces shredded cheddar cheese blend
- 1 bag riced cauliflower
- 4 tablespoons butter
- ¼ cup Buffalo sauce
- ½ cup ranch dressing
- 1 teaspoon minced garlic
- ¼ teaspoon sea salt + additional for seasoning
- Black pepper
- Garlic powder
- Nonstick cooking spray

Directions:

- Preheat oven to 350.
- Spray baking dish with nonstick spray.
- Season chicken with salt, pepper and garlic powder on both sides.
- Layer chicken onto baking dish.
- Place in oven for 15 minutes.
- In a separate saucepan, melt butter and garlic together over low heat.
- Once butter is melted, remove from heat.
- Stir in Buffalo sauce, ranch dressing, salt and pepper. Stir to combine. (Add ¼ teaspoon cayenne pepper for extra spice).
- After 15 minutes, remove chicken from oven.
- Add cauliflower rice into baking dish. Place on sides of chicken or in between.
- Pour sauce over chicken and rice. Top with cheese.
- Bake for additional 15-20 minutes, or until cheese is melted and chicken reaches an internal temperature of 165.

Lazy Gourmet

Crock-pot

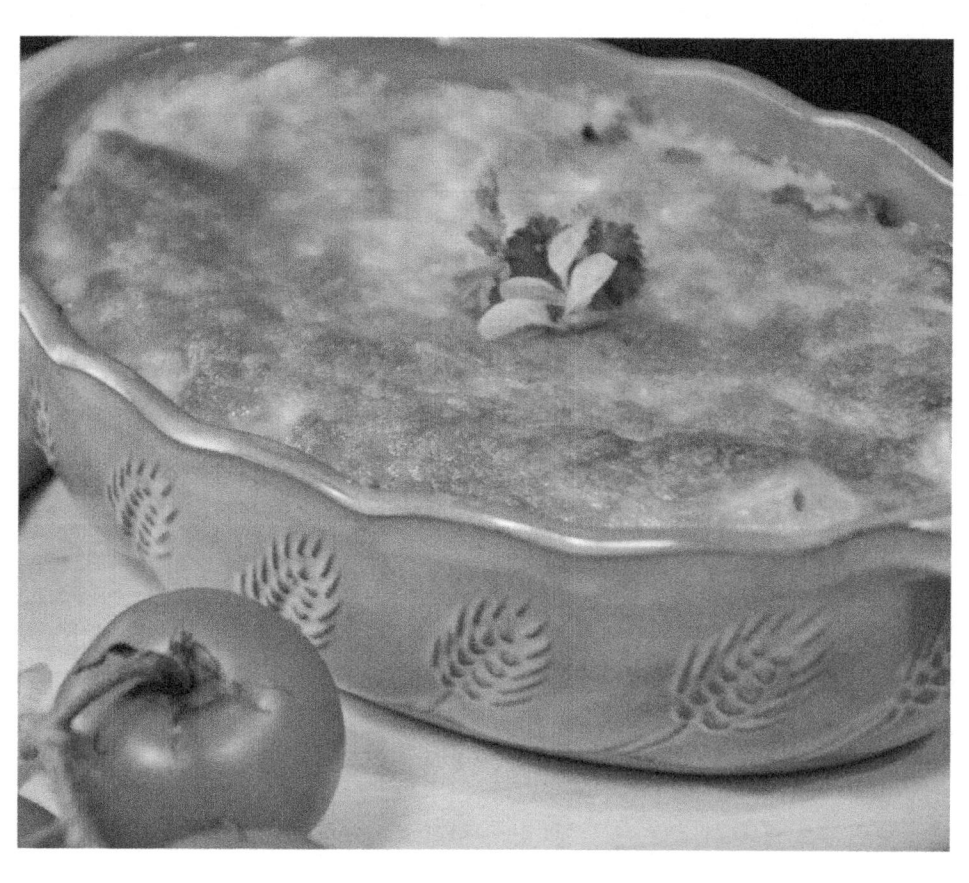

Lazy Gourmet Crock-Pot

What can be lazier than crock-pot meals? What can be tastier than *The Lazy Keto Gourmet* crock-pot meals? Very little is your answer.

When I cook crock-pot meals, I cook large batches so I have leftovers to heat up during the week for lunch or for an easy dinner when my husband travels. You can even freeze leftovers and take them out when you are ready for a quick meal. Most of the recipes I list will serve a family of four. Keep in mind I am a mere stay-at-home mom, so I do not dare take a stab at what the normal family of four considers a serving size. My husband and I eat large servings and we always have leftovers. That's as scientific as I get here.

When you prepare your meal, don't forget to spray the crock-pot with a nonstick spray for easier clean up. I use a coconut oil based spray because coconut oil is a great oil for withstanding heat. Not all oils are great when heated. Here's looking at you olive oil.

Do not keep opening the lid while you are cooking. Everytime you open that lid, you extend cooking time.

If you want more crock-pot cooking tips, check out *The KETO Crock-pot Cookbook* by Carrie Brown. She has great tips and delicious recipes. That is where I found the barbeque sauce I use for the recipes in this book. It is the best barbeque sauce I've had; low-carb or otherwise.

Shredded Chicken & Bacon Alfredo

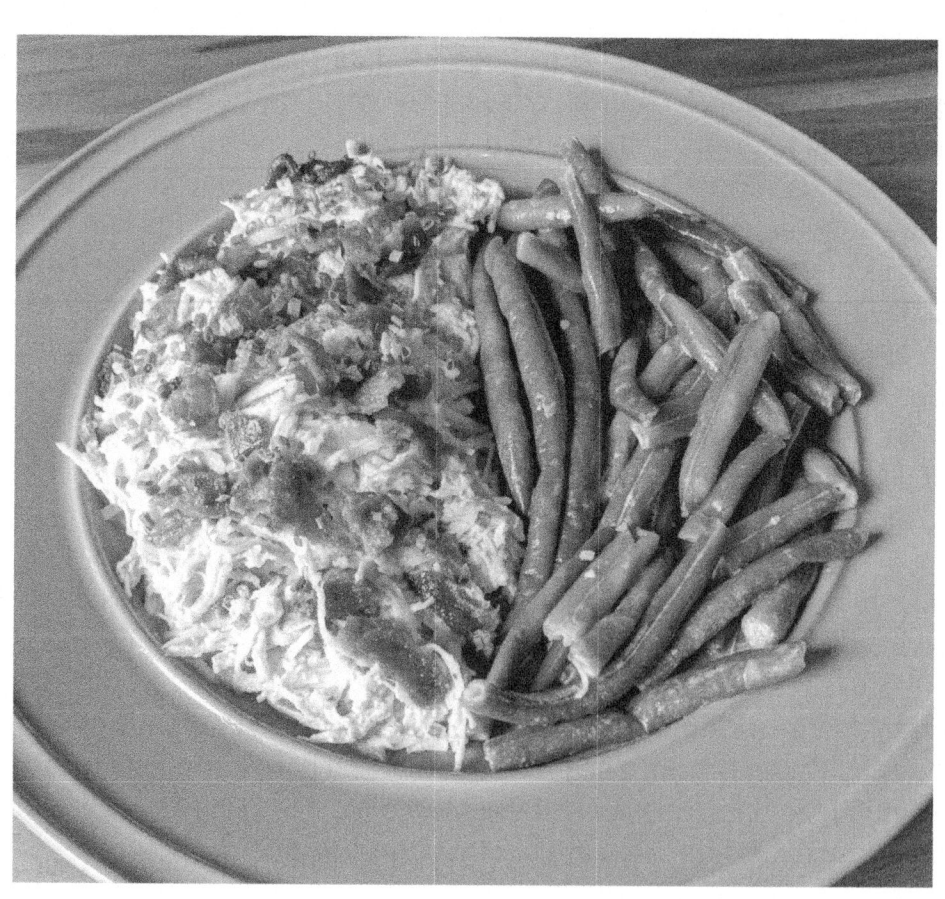

Ingredients:

- 2 pounds chicken breasts or thighs
- 2 tablespoons butter
- 1 teaspoon minced garlic
- 2 cups heavy cream
- ½ pound bacon, cooked and crumbled into bacon bits
- Green onions, chopped
- Sea salt
- Black pepper
- Nonstick cooking spray

Directions:

- Spray crock-pot with nonstick spray.
- Season both sides of chicken with black pepper and salt. Place in crock-pot.
- In saucepan, melt butter and minced garlic together. Cook on low for approximately 2-3 minutes, or until butter is melted.
- Add heavy cream to saucepan. Heat for few minutes while whisking together the cream, butter and garlic. Once combined, pour over chicken.
- Cook on low for 4-6 hours.
- Shred chicken with 2 forks or hand mixer. Add in bacon bits and stir.
- Garnish with chopped green onions.

Crock-Pot
Buffalo Chicken

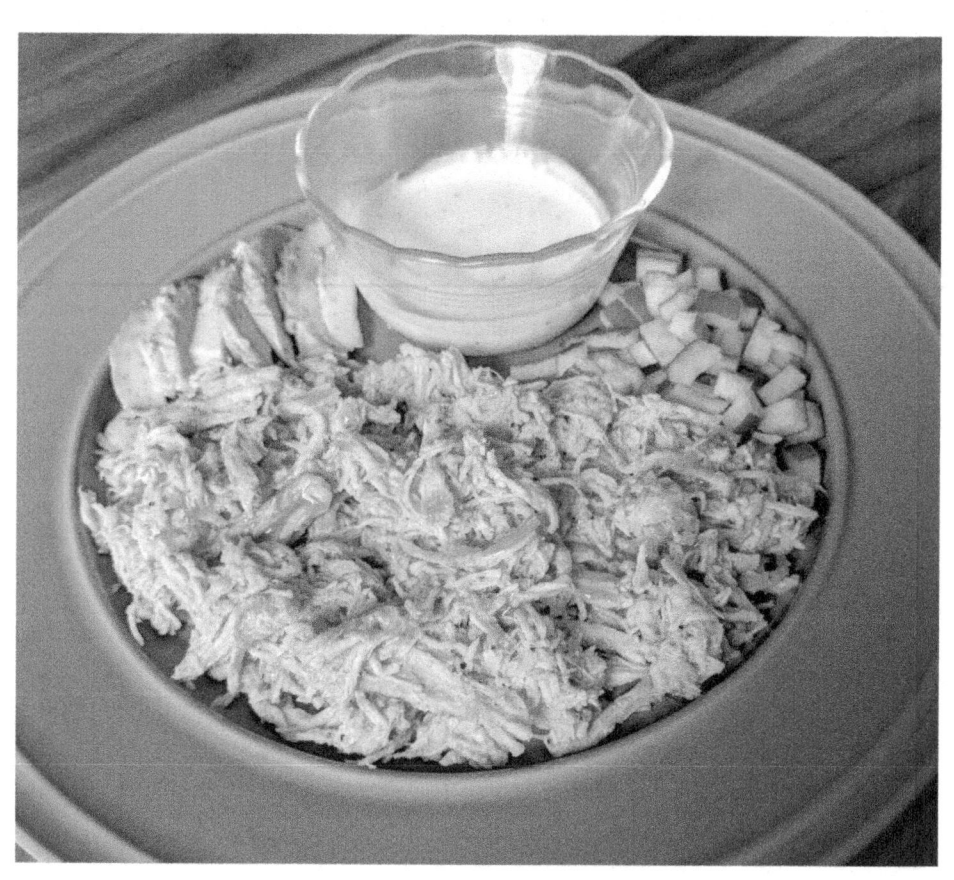

Ingredients:

- Two pounds chicken thighs or breasts
- 12 ounces Buffalo sauce
- 4 – 8 tablespoons butter
- Powdered garlic
- Black pepper
- Nonstick cooking spray

Directions:

- Spray crock-pot with nonstick cooking spray.
- Season boneless chicken thighs or breasts with garlic powder and black pepper on both sides.
- Place chicken into crock-pot and pour Buffalo sauce over chicken.
- Cook on low for 7-8 hours or high for 3-4 hours.
- Once cooked, add in butter.
- Allow butter to melt as you shred chicken with two large forks or with a hand mixer on low.
- Stir and serve with your favorite toppings. Mine include red onions, avocado and ranch.

Chicken Avocado Salad

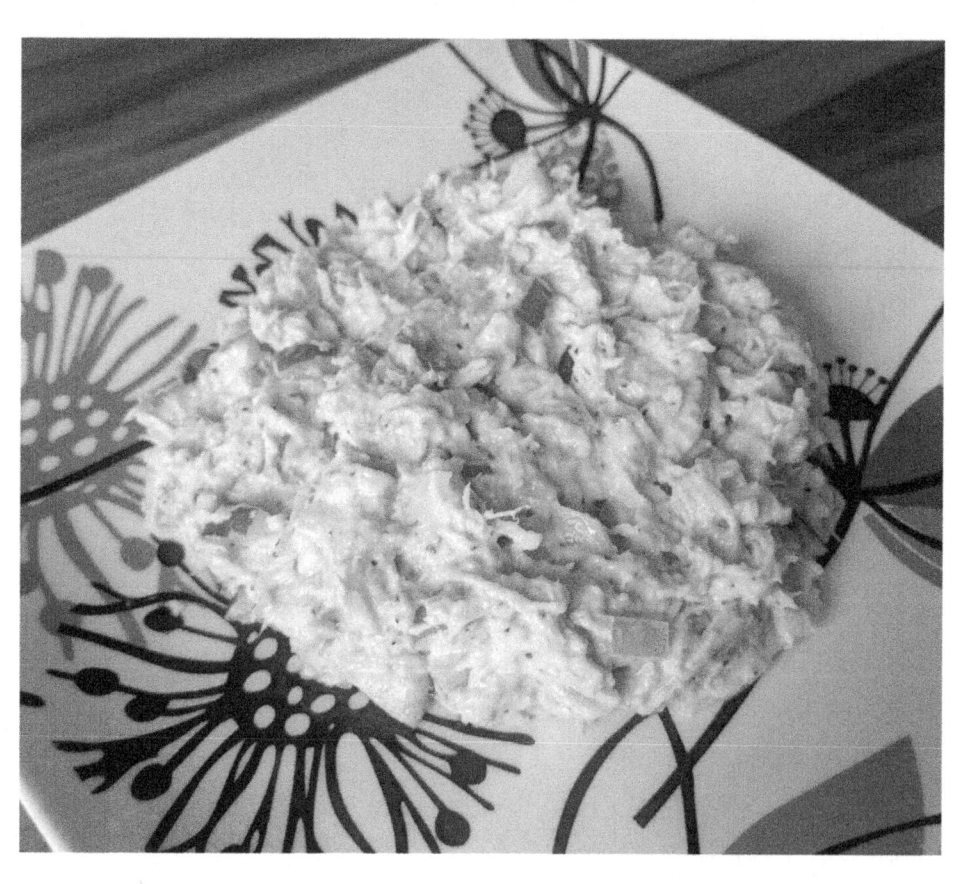

Ingredients:

- 1 pound chicken breasts or thighs
- 1 cup chicken broth
- 1 avocado, chopped
- 1 cup bacon crumbles
- ½ - 1 cup full fat mayonnaise
- 1 small red onion, chopped
- 1 teaspoon minced garlic
- ½ teaspoon black pepper + extra to season chicken
- ⅛ - ¼ teaspoon red pepper flakes
- Garlic powder
- 2 teaspoons lime juice
- Nonstick cooking spray

Directions:

- Spray crock-pot with nonstick spray.
- Pour chicken broth into crock-pot.
- Season both sides of chicken with pepper and garlic powder to taste.
- Layer chicken on top of chicken broth in crock-pot.
- Cook for 3-4 hours on high or 7-8 hours on low.
- Shred chicken with two forks. Allow chicken to cool in fridge for 30 minutes.
- Add cooled chicken, bacon crumbles, avocado, onions, minced garlic, lime juice, red pepper flakes and mayo into a large mixing bowl. Combine.
- Serve immediately or place in fridge. Serve cold.

Sweet & Tangy BBQ Chicken

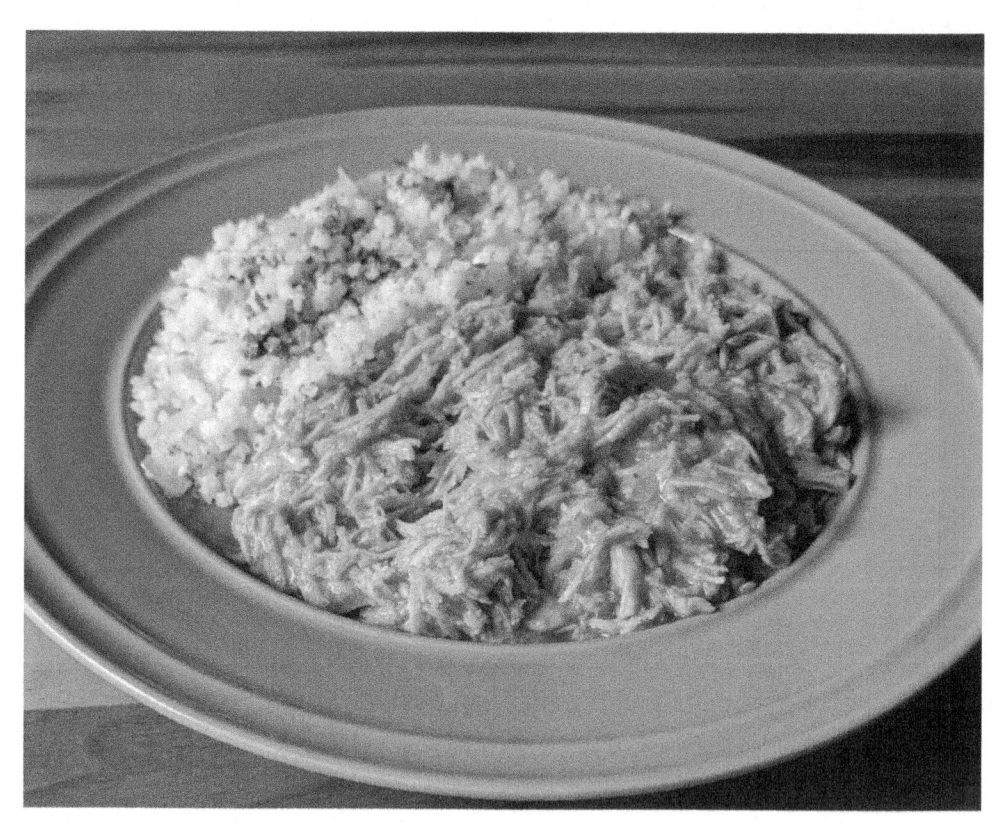

Ingredients:

- 2 pounds chicken breasts or thighs
- 12 ounces low sugar BBQ sauce
- ½ cup Italian salad dressing
- 2 tablespoons worcestershire sauce
- Salt, pepper and garlic powder to season chicken
- 4 tablespoons butter
- Nonstick cooking spray

Directions:

- Spray crock-pot with nonstick cooking spray.
- Season chicken with salt, pepper and garlic powder to taste.
- Layer chicken breasts or thighs into crock-pot.
- In mixing bowl, combine low sugar BBQ sauce, Italian salad dressing and worcestershire sauce.
- Pour sauce over chicken.
- Cover. Cook on high for 3-4 hours or low for 4-6 hours.
- Once cooked, add butter to crock-pot.
- While butter melts, shred chicken with two forks or with a hand mixer on low.
- Stir and serve.

Lazy Gourmet

Favorites

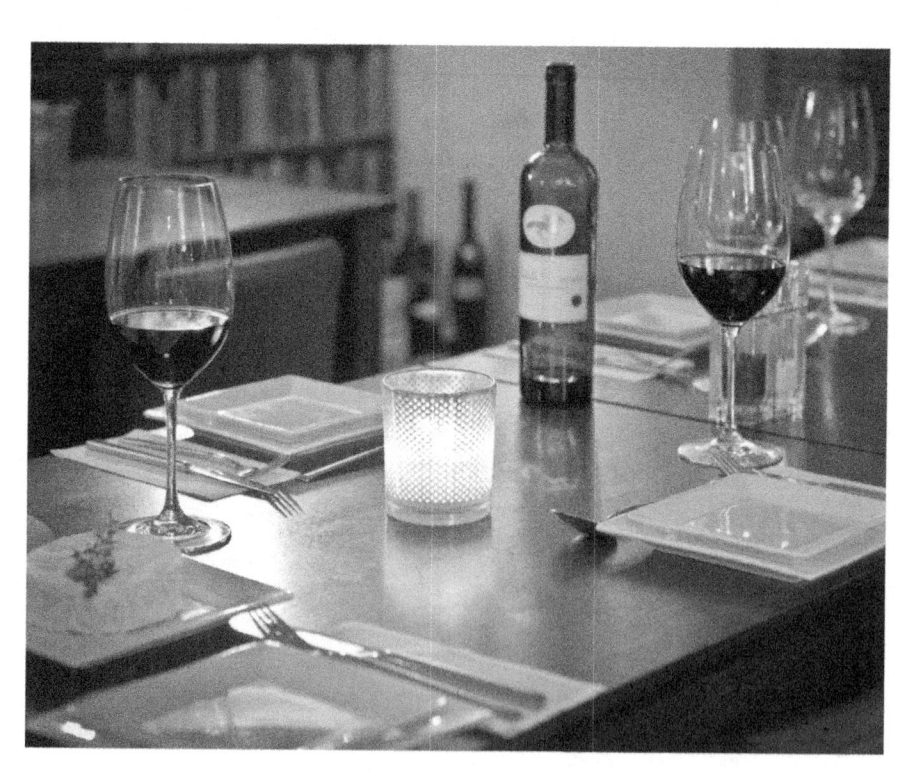

Lazy Gourmet Favorites

While this is the shortest section of the book, it very well may be the most important. This section contains my favorite go-to meals! I make these meals as often as I possibly can. I really cannot get enough.

The exception is the sausage crust pizza. I. Love. Pizza. I could live on pizza alone. Unfortunately pizza does not love me. When I eat too much cheese, I notice my nose starts to drip soon after consumption. The next morning I wake up with a scratchy throat at a minimum. Upon maximum cheese overload, I wake up with full on cheese flu. I feel achy and like my throat is on fire.

I also noticed an increase in painful acne before I improved my digestion. Now I only feel a small pimple forming upon consumption of too much cream cheese. All of this means I have to save up my cheese binges as an every once in a while treat. Darn you cheese! Why must you be so delicious?

The reason I have these symptoms is I am sensitive to the casein protein in cheese and other dairy. That means I can eat all of the butter I want since it is mostly fat, but when it comes to the melty stuff and other dairy products, I limit my consumption to avoid feeling bad the next day. Sometimes we have to sacrifice for health. Sometimes those sacrifices come in the form of avoiding food made from the curds of milk.

There are other reasons you too may want to limit your dairy. The sugar in cheese is called lactose. For some unlucky individuals, consumption of lactose causes constipation. For other sensitive individuals, eating cheese can keep them out of ketosis and stall their weight loss completely because of the lactose. These are all things you need to test and make the best decision for the lifestyle you want. If you want to squeeze baseball sized poops out everyday because you *need* the gooey stuff, that's all you. I had the baseball sized poops two times after having my children. #neveragain

Another alternative is to add digestive enzymes to your supplement protocol to help your body digest lactose. More specifically, you can add Milk Gest enzymes to your meals with dairy. These contain the lactase enzyme. Your body could be missing that and supplementing with this when you eat dairy could be just the thing you need to have your cheese and eat it too!

I use Milk Gest found on naturalreference.com to help with my digestion of dairy. If you order, please use my practitioner code at checkout: nissahelpsme. You can seek out other brands, but I cannot attest to their quality since I have only used Milk Gest.

Sausage Crust Pizza

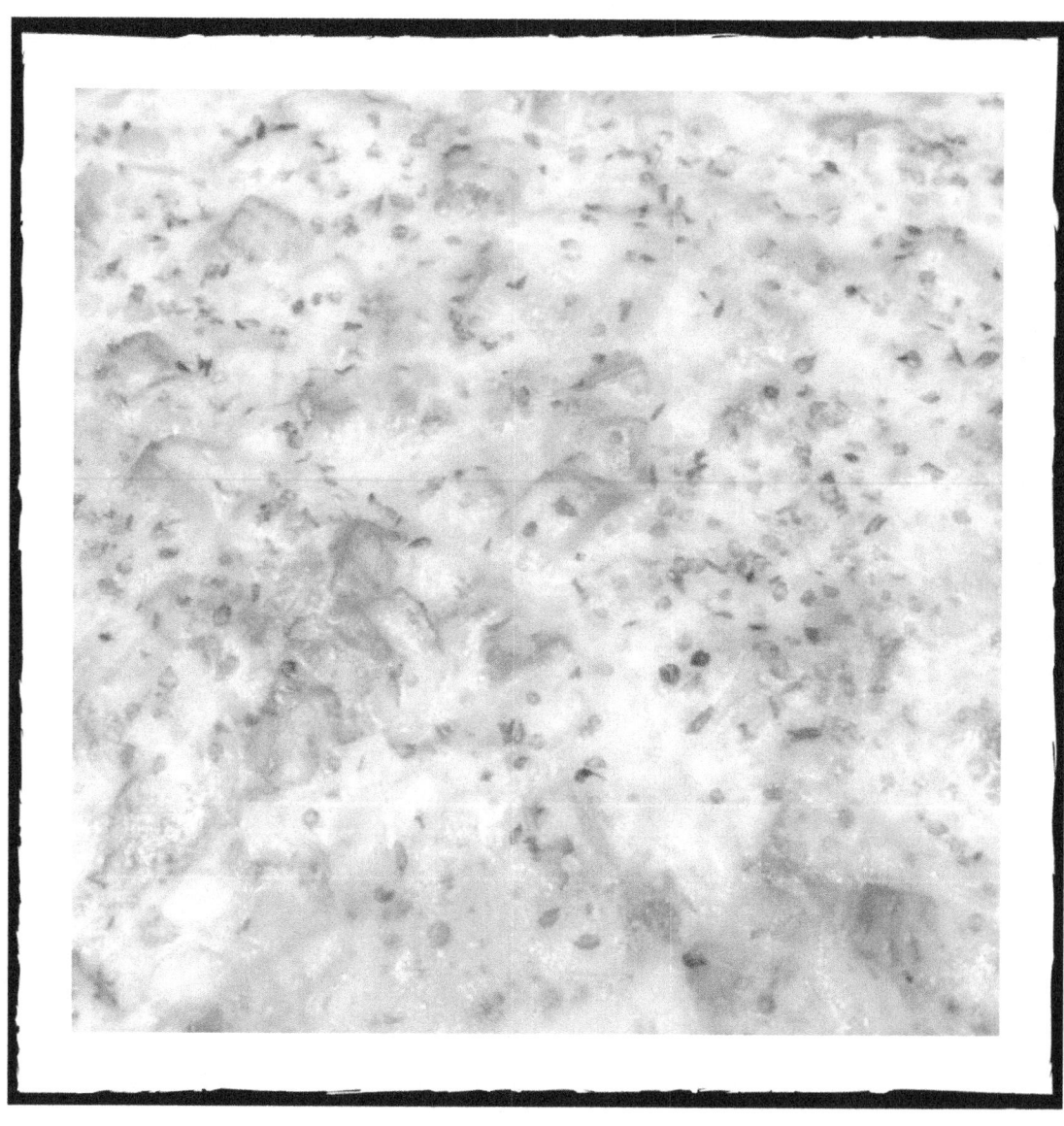

Ingredients:

- 1 pound ground Italian sausage
- 1 cup low-carb marinara sauce
- 6 ounces shredded mozzarella cheese
- 2 teaspoons garlic powder
- 1 tablespoon and ½ teaspoon Italian seasoning
- ½ tablespoon minced garlic
- ¼ teaspoon salt
- ¼ teaspoon pepper
- 1 teaspoon oregano + extra to sprinkle

Directions:

- Preheat oven to 350 degrees.
- On an ungreased pan, flatten sausage with hands or rolling pin to form crust.
- Sprinkle with garlic powder and 1 tablespoon of Italian seasoning.
- Place in oven for 20 minutes, or until crust is mostly cooked.
- In mixing bowl, add marinara sauce, ½ teaspoon Italian seasoning, oregano, minced garlic, salt and black pepper. Stir well.
- Remove partially cooked crust from oven. Layer sauce on top.
- Layer additional ingredients. I add diced onion, diced green pepper and pepperoni.
- Layer cheese on top. Sprinkle with oregano.
- Place in oven until cheese is melted, approximately 10 – 12 minutes.
- Slice and enjoy!

Bacon Avocado & Cucumber Salad

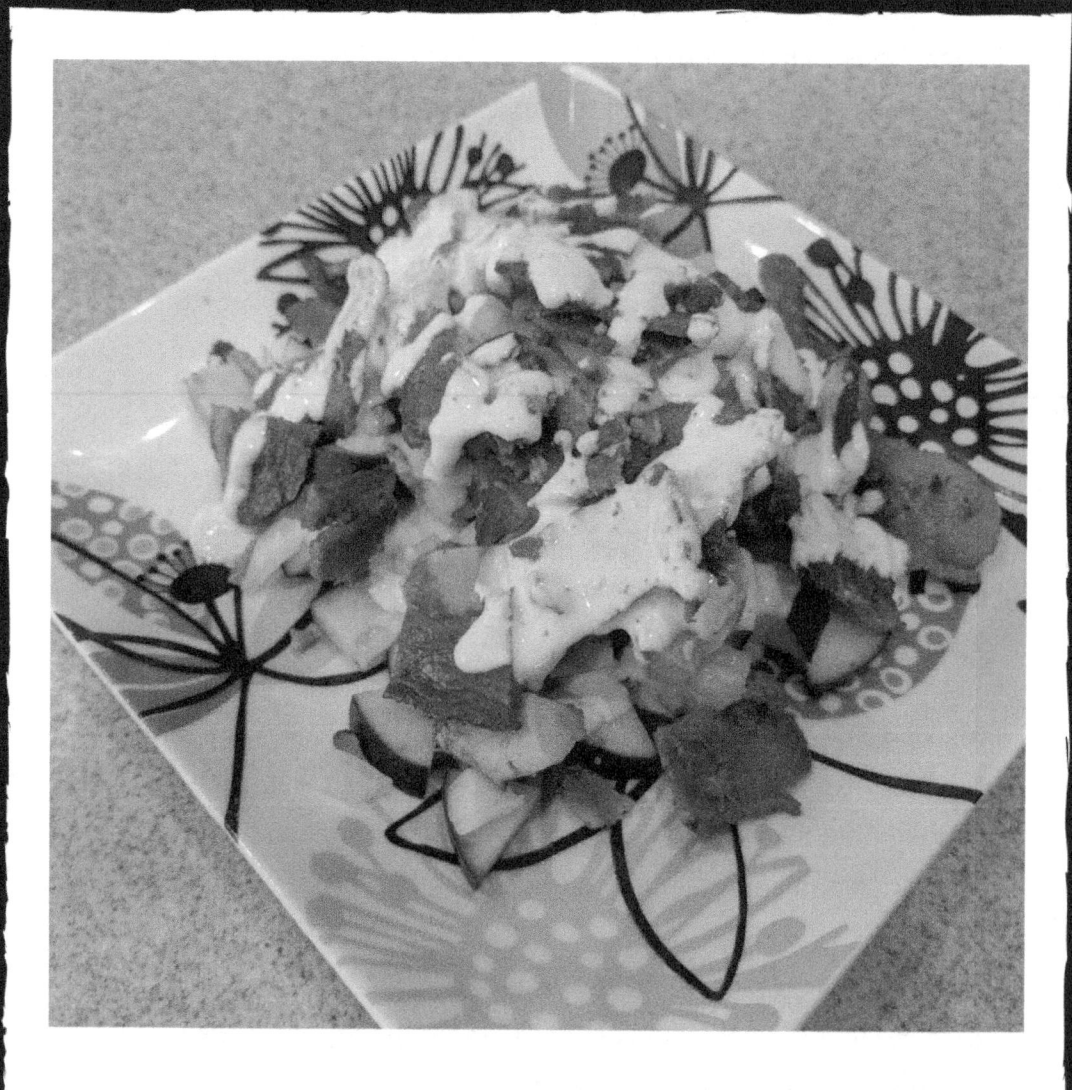

Ingredients:

- 3 ounces bacon, cooked
- 4 ounces cucumbers
- ½ avocado
- ½ ounce red onion
- 1 ounce ranch salad dressing

Directions:

- Chop bacon, cucumbers, avocado and onion.
- Layer cucumbers, avocado, onions, and chopped bacon on plate.
- Drizzle ranch over salad.
- Enjoy!

*TIP: I cook bacon in large batches and keep in the fridge for up to a week.

Mediterranean Steak Strips

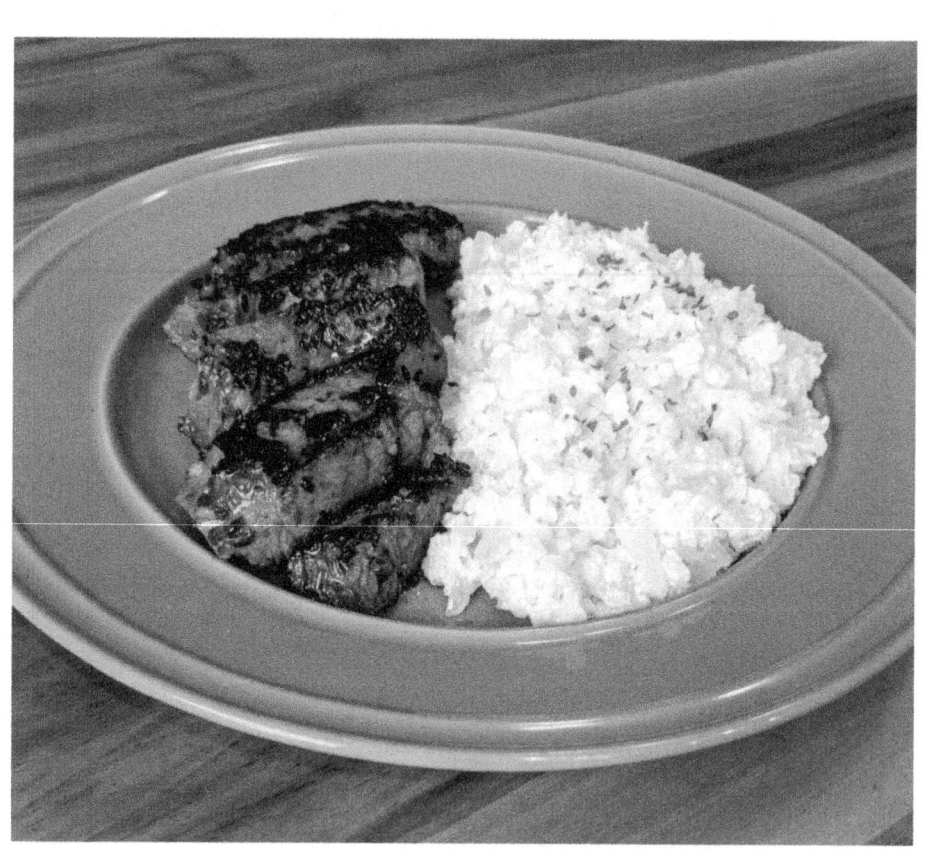

Ingredients:

- 1 pound steak of choice
- ⅓ cup olive oil
- ¼ cup coconut aminos
- ¼ cup worcestershire sauce
- 2 teaspoons minced garlic
- 2 tablespoons dried basil
- 1 tablespoon oregano
- 1 teaspoon black pepper

Directions:

- Cut steak into 1 inch thick strips.
- Place all ingredients (except steak) in a ziploc bag. Close and shake bag to mix marinade.
- Place steak in ziploc bag and shake gently to coat steak.
- Let steak marinate for 4-24 hours in fridge.
- Heat a large skillet over medium-high heat until it is very hot. With tongs, remove steak from bag and place into skillet.
- Cook steak for 3 minutes per side for a medium temperature.

Lazy Gourmet

Ground Beef

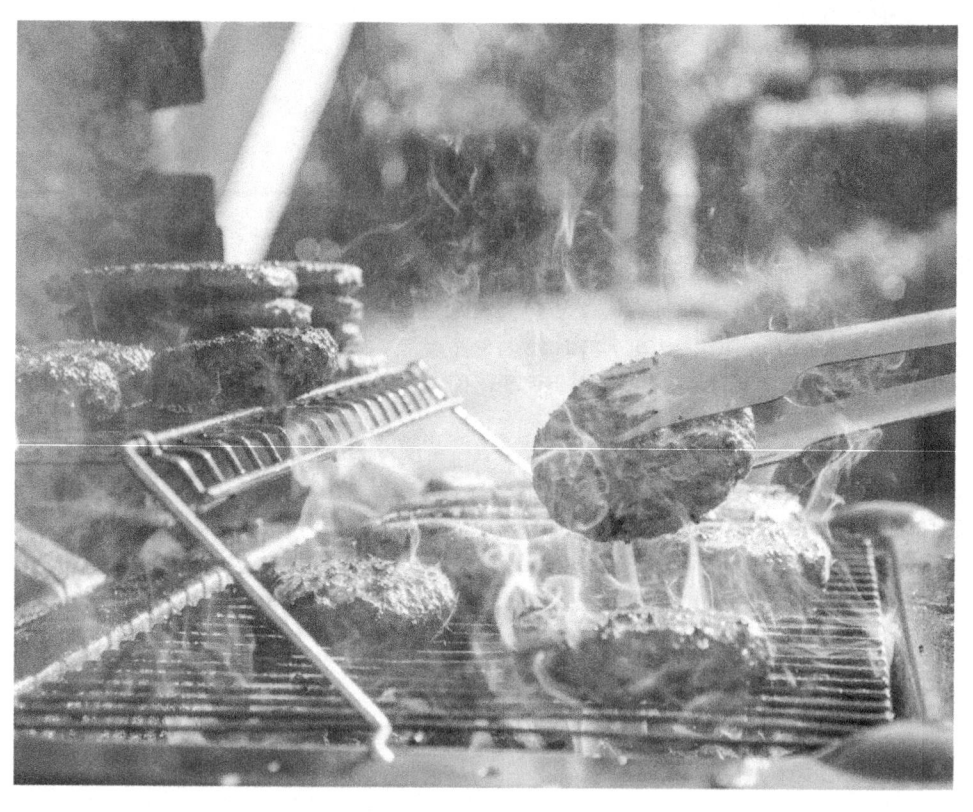

Lazy Gourmet Ground Beef

Please take a second to review the title of this section. Ground beef. Ground beef is not the same thing as ground turkey. I understand Weight Watchers taught you to make this easy substitution for lower points. Weight Watchers also stomped your thriving metabolism into the ground, so let's reset.

If you prefer ground turkey to higher fat ground beef, this is a digestion problem. You can tell me all you want that you prefer the taste. No one with properly functioning digestion prefers ground turkey to high fat ground beef. If you think you do, work on digesting high quality proteins and fats for a while and then give both meats a blindfolded taste test. You will gag on the ground turkey.

With a low-carb, high-fat diet, you want to focus on eating high-fat foods to heal your hormones. Ground turkey is not a high-fat food. It is a low-calorie, low-taste substitution. Same thing goes for turkey bacon, in case that part isn't obvious.

If you are not digesting proteins well, you need to enroll in the digestion course. I get it. I was there for a few months after my first pregnancy. I could no longer stomach a juicy steak. Whenever I tried, it tasted like raw cow and made me extremely nauseous. This did not improve until I began to supplement with Beatine HCL. This was due in large part to all of the Tums I took for the massive heartburn I had during pregnancy. Taking antacids killed my stomach acid, as is their intent. When you do not have proper stomach acid to break down high quality proteins, your food can taste like raw cow.

There are many other reasons you want properly functioning stomach acid. If you have any of the following symptoms, your stomach acid could use some work: heartburn, low blood pressure, burping, undigested food in your stool, constipation or difficulty losing weight. If you do not have sufficient stomach acid, your food is not being broken down properly. If your food is not being broken down properly, you are not getting the nutrients you are eating. This leads to poor health and accumulation of unwanted fat rolls.

So we talked about choosing ground beef over turkey. Along those same lines, let's choose high quality meats too. Organic, grass fed meats are always going to be your best option. These contain the best nutrients. Cows that eat the foods they are not meant to eat that have also been sprayed with pesticides do not contain the best nutrients. These are sick cows. Sick cows make cheap meat. Cheap meat makes sick humans.

When I speak of choosing higher quality, I also mean choosing higher fat ground beef too. Don't make me lecture you about Weight Watchers all over again. If you are not yet able to digest higher fat meat, get the lower fat stuff for now while you work on your digestion. Work up to the higher fat meat as your body is better able to process it. Don't be complacent and settle for low-fat, low quality food forever. Do the work.

I would like to add in a word of warning about the ground beef recipes. Some of them also contain extra fats like butter since butter melted on beef tastes surprisingly good. Some people even use a butter and beef fast to break a weight loss stall. I'm not sure of the magical logic there, but that is one fast that is not meant for this girl. I would rather avoid food completely to break my stall. I am referring to intermittent fasting, not anorexia, in this case.

The reason I bring up the butter or other added fats in the beef recipes goes back to digestion. If you are not digesting fats well, do not attempt to add too many extra fats to the beef recipes. Leave them out since ground beef is higher in fat than chicken. The recipes still work without the extra fats in most recipes. I have long since improved my digestion, yet sometimes the addition of butter to the sweet & spicy spaghetti sauce is still too much for me. It is a tasty addition if you can handle that much fat, but proceed with caution if you cannot.

Spicy Burgers

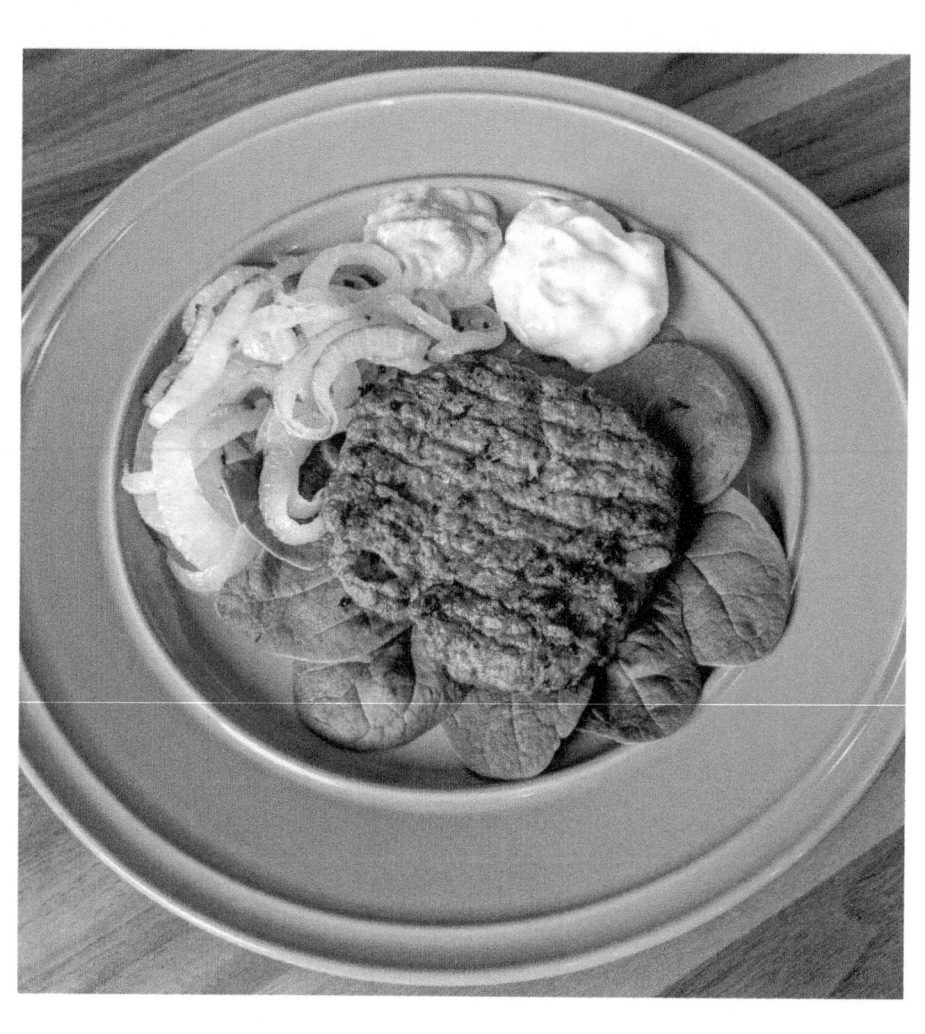

Ingredients:

- 1 and ⅓ pounds 80% ground beef
- ⅓ cup onions, finely chopped
- ¼ cup worcestershire sauce
- 2 teaspoons minced garlic
- ¼ – ½ teaspoon red pepper flakes
- ½ teaspoon pepper
- ½ teaspoon salt

Directions:

- Mix all ingredients in mixing bowl with hands.
- Form burgers into patties with hands or burger press. Recipe makes 4-5 burgers.
- Grill or pan fry to desired temp.
- Top with cheese, bacon, grilled onions, avocado slices, mayo or other toppings of choice.

Tip: Coconut sauteed onions is an easy and tasty addition to spicy burgers.

The Mac Salad

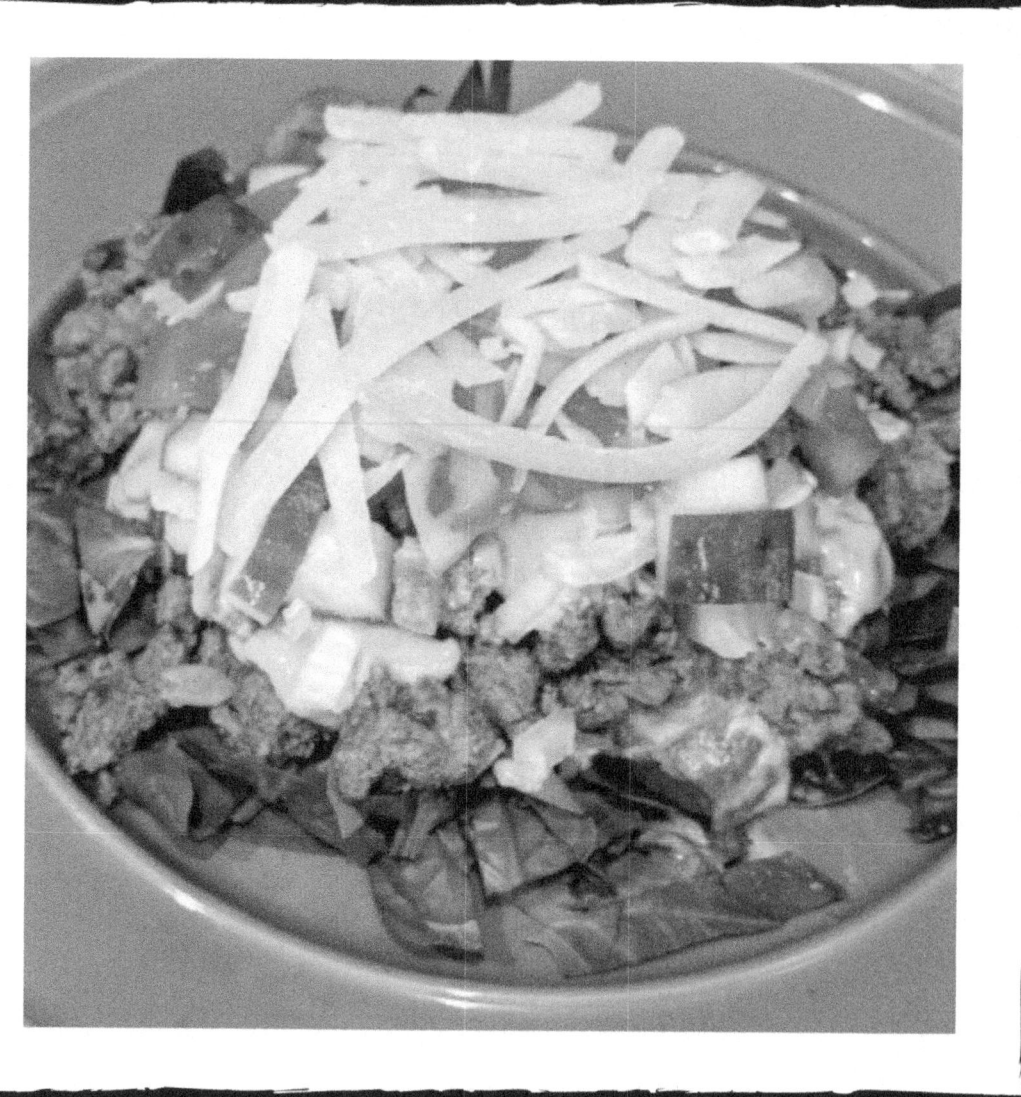

Ingredients:

- 1 pound 80% ground beef
- 4 ounces shredded cheddar cheese
- 4-6 cups chopped spinach
- 1 and ½ cups finely chopped onion
- Small tomato, chopped
- 1 teaspoon minced garlic
- ½ teaspoon onion powder
- Sea salt & black pepper to taste
- 3 tablespoons yellow mustard
- Whole pickle, chopped
- 4-6 ounces Thousand Island dressing

Directions:

- Brown ground beef in large skillet.
- Add 1 cup finely chopped onions, minced garlic, onion powder, salt and pepper to ground beef while it is browning.
- Once beef is browned, remove skillet from heat. Mix in 3 tablespoons yellow mustard. Stir well.
- Layer Big Mac Salad on plate:
    - Chopped spinach
    - ½ serving Thousand Island dressing
    - Ground beef mixture
    - ½ serving Thousand Island dressing
    - Pickles, tomatoes & remaining chopped onions
    - Cheddar cheese

*Recipe makes approximately 4 servings. Make one large salad or plate separately.

Buffalo Ranch Taco Salad

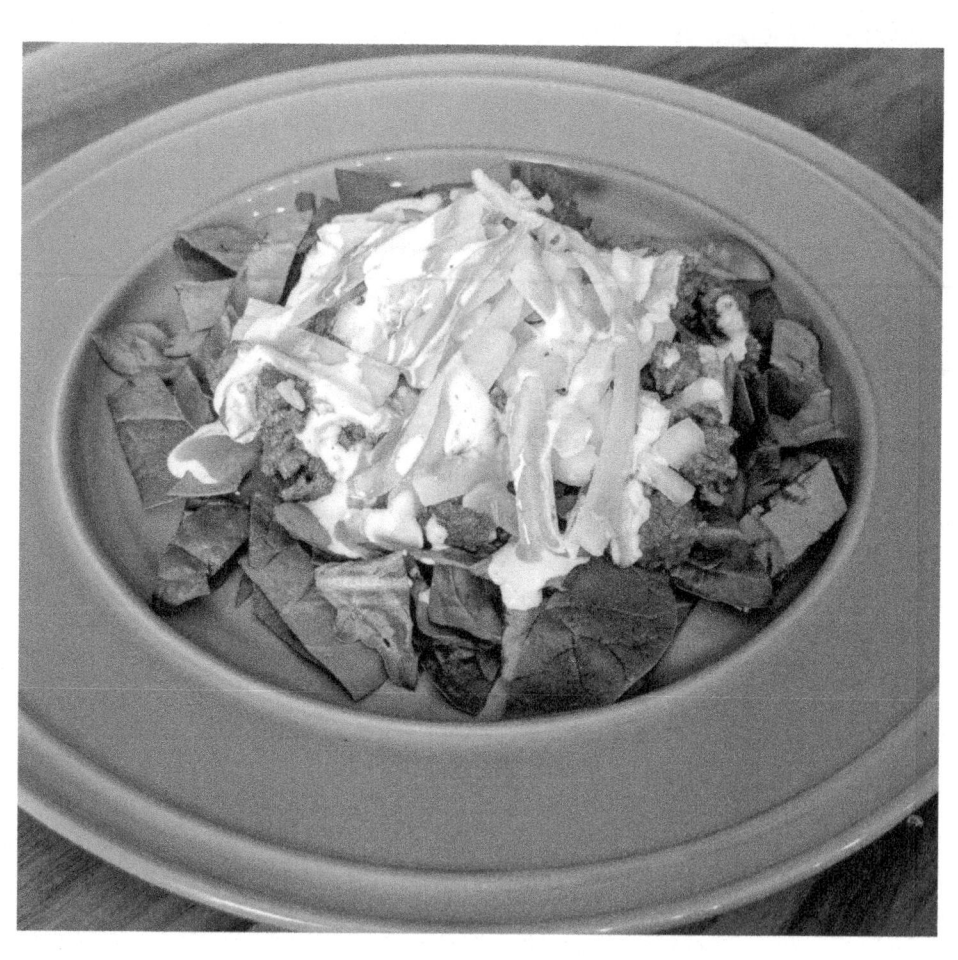

Ingredients:

- 1 pound 80% ground beef
- 1 packet taco seasoning
- 2 teaspoons minced garlic
- ¾ cup water
- 4 ounces ranch dressing
- 2 ounces Buffalo sauce
- 4-6 cups spinach, chopped
- 1 yellow onion, chopped
- 1 tomato, chopped
- 4 ounces shredded Mexican cheese

Directions:

- Brown ground beef in skillet.
- Add minced garlic while browning beef.
- Once browned, stir in taco seasoning and water.
- Bring to a boil; then simmer for 5 minutes.
- Allow beef to cool.
- In a large bowl, combine beef, lettuce, onion, tomato, cheese, Buffalo sauce and ranch. Toss until evenly coated.
- Serve immediately. Alternatively, this can be served cold from the fridge.

Layered Taco Salad

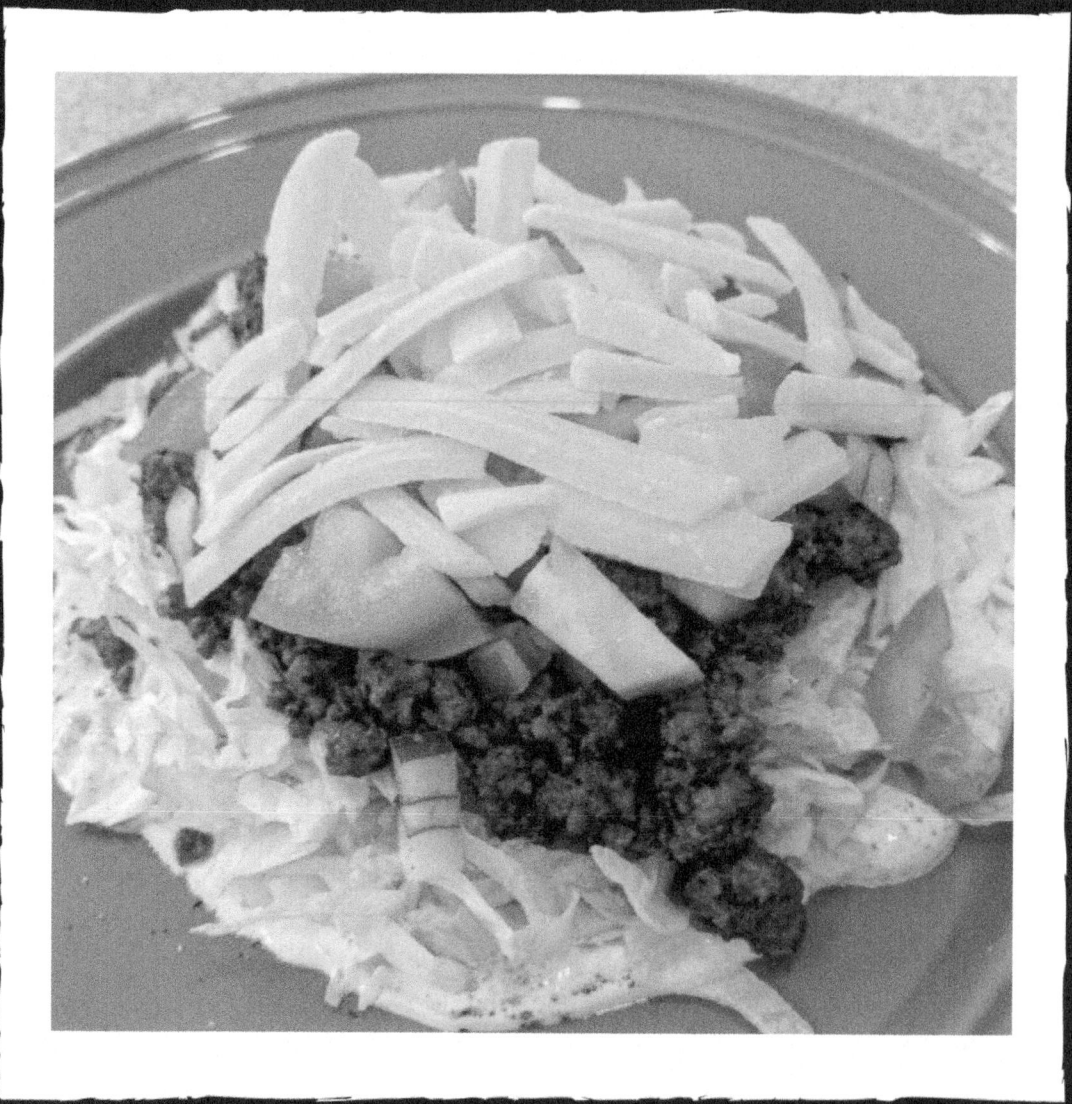

Ingredients:

- 1 pound 80% ground beef
- 1 and ½ ounces taco seasoning
- ¾ cup water
- 4 ounces sour cream
- 4 ounces shredded cheddar cheese
- 1 tomato, chopped
- 1 small red onion, chopped
- 1 bag shredded lettuce

Directions:

- Brown ground beef in skillet.
- Once browned, stir in 1 ounce taco seasoning and ¾ cup of water. Bring to boil, then reduce to simmer for 5-10 minutes.
- Allow ground beef to cool slightly.
- Layer serving plate with sour cream. Stir remaining taco seasoning into sour cream.
- Top sour cream with shredded lettuce, ground beef, chopped onion, chopped tomatoes and shredded cheese.

*Recipe makes approximately 4 servings. Make one large salad or plate separately.

Sweet & Spicy Spaghetti Sauce

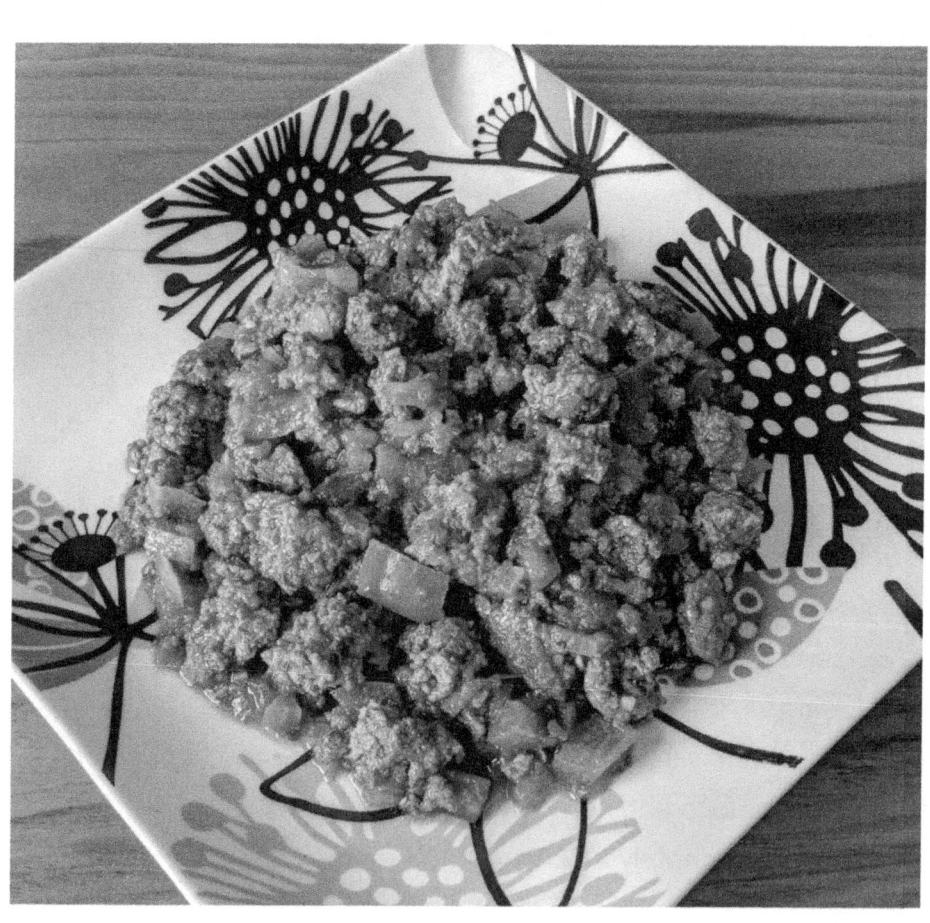

Ingredients:

- 1 pound 80% ground beef
- 1 jar low-carb marinara sauce
- 2 tablespoons butter
- 2 tablespoons olive oil
- 2 teaspoons minced garlic
- 1 small sweet onion, chopped
- 1 green pepper, chopped
- 1 teaspoon cinnamon
- Oregano
- Crushed red pepper

Directions:

- Brown ground beef in large skillet.
- While browning, season with oregano and add crushed red pepper to taste. Stir in onions, green peppers and minced garlic.
- Once meat is browned, turn heat to medium-low.
- Add butter. As butter melts, add jar of marinara sauce and stir.
- Sprinkle cinnamon over sauce.
- Remove from heat. Stir in olive oil.
- Mix well and serve.

Creamy & Spicy Spaghetti Sauce

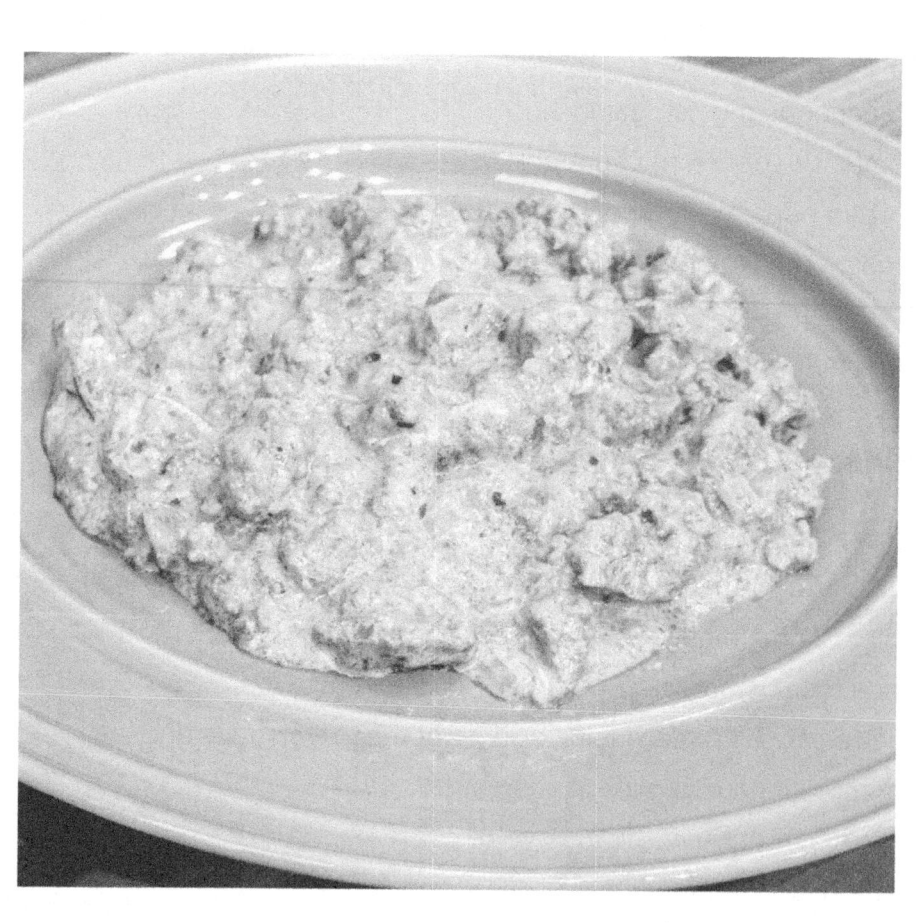

Ingredients:

- 1 pound 80% ground beef
- 1 cup low sugar marinara sauce
- 1 cup heavy whipping cream
- 2 tablespoons butter
- 1 sweet onion, chopped
- 1 green pepper, chopped
- 3 teaspoons minced garlic, divided
- Crushed red pepper
- Italian seasoning

Directions:

- Melt 2 tablespoons butter over low heat in saucepan.
- Once melted stir in 2 teaspoons minced garlic until lightly browned, or 2-3 minutes.
- Once garlic browns, add ½ cup heavy cream to saucepan.
- Stir frequently until sauce thickens (5-10 minutes).
- Repeat with remaining ½ cup heavy cream.
- Once sauce thickens, add marinara sauce. Stir well.

While Cooking Sauce:

- Brown ground beef in skillet.
- While beef is browning, add 1 teaspoon minced garlic and season with Italian seasoning and crushed red pepper to taste. Stir in diced onion and green pepper.
- Once browned, pour thickened sauce over beef mixture.
- Stir and serve.

Buffalo Ranch Meatballs

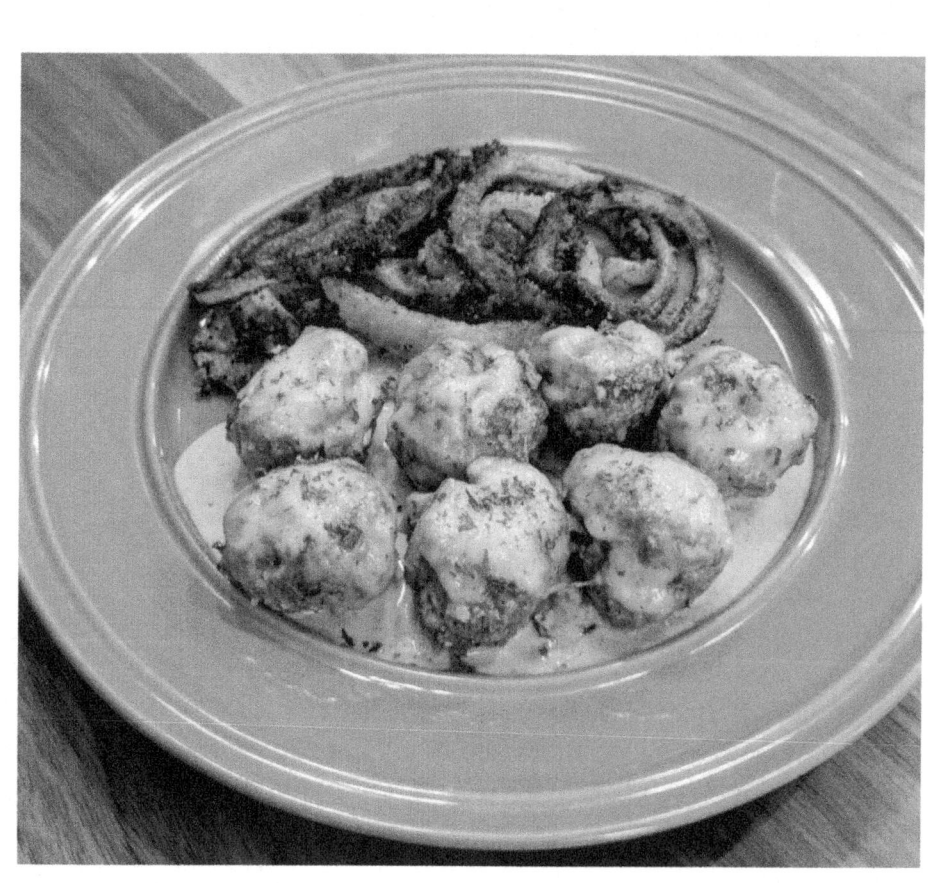

Ingredients:

- 1 ⅓ pounds 80% ground beef
- 2 tablespoons fresh parsley, chopped
- ½ cup almond flour
- 3 teaspoons minced garlic
- 1 teaspoon salt
- ¼ teaspoon black pepper
- 1 teaspoon onion flakes
- ½ teaspoon oregano
- ½ cup water, room temperature
- 2-3 tablespoons coconut oil
- 4 ounces swiss cheese
- ½ cup ranch dressing
- ¼ cup Buffalo sauce
- Nonstick cooking spray

Directions:

- Preheat oven to 350 degrees.
- Spray baking dish with nonstick spray.
- Add ground beef, parsley, almond flour, 2 teaspoons minced garlic, salt, pepper, onion flakes, oregano and water in a mixing bowl. Mix ingredients with hands.
- Form meatballs into 2 inch balls with hands.
- Heat coconut oil in large skillet on high heat.
- Fry meatballs in coconut oil until lightly browned, 2-3 minutes per side.
- Add meatballs to baking dish.
- Combine ranch dressing, 1 teaspoon minced garlic and Buffalo sauce in bowl.
- Pour half of the Buffalo ranch sauce over the meatballs.
- Layer swiss cheese on top.
- Bake in oven for 15-20 minutes.
- Garnish with extra parsley.
- Layer leftover Buffalo ranch sauce on plate. Add meatballs on top.

Sauces & Sides

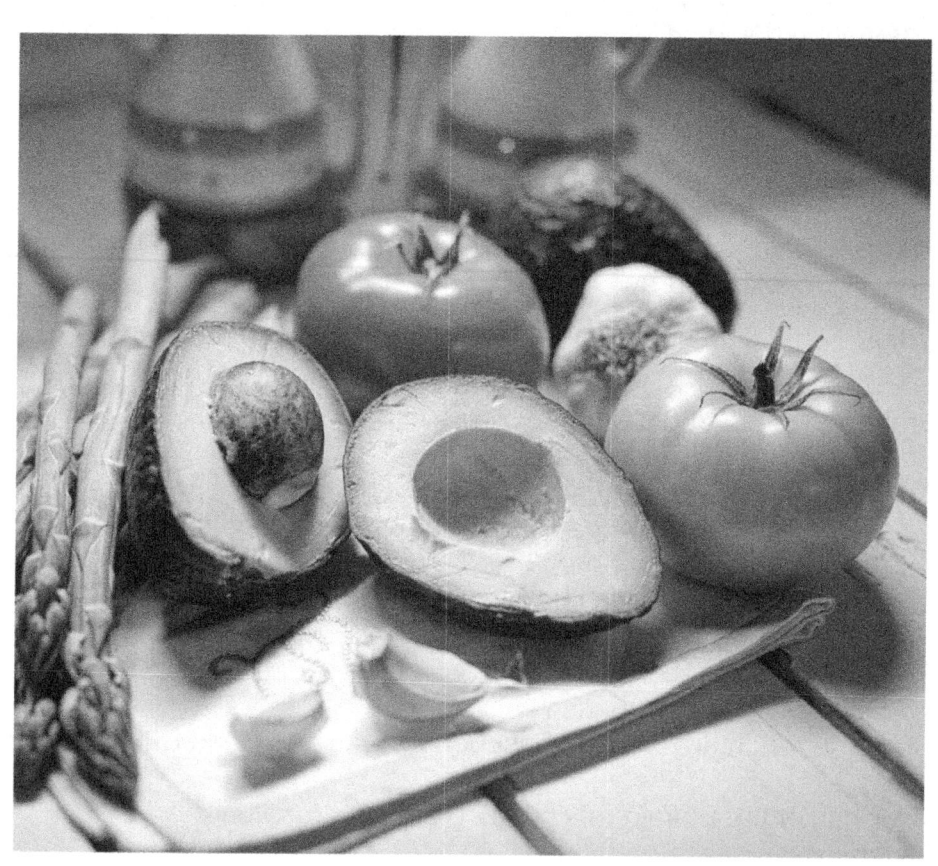

Sauces & Sides

This section is going to be less about teaching and more about tips on obtaining the best results with the sauces and sides. If you are hooked on the teaching aspect of this cookbook, don't forget about that six week course I put together: Escape Diet Mentality and End Yo-Yo Diets Forever. You receive emails every day for six full weeks. The teaching in the course is endless! Except it ends after six weeks.

Rich, creamy sauces are going to be one of the easiest ways to add extra fat into your diet without adding a lot of extra protein or carbs. This is important when you are following a ketogenic diet. If you are adhering to less strict low-carb, high-fat logic, not quite as important, but still tasty.

Unlike those in the keto crowd who tell you to limit fat on a high-fat diet, that's not how this works. That's not how any of this works. These people tell you if you have fat to burn on your body, taking in more healthy fats is going to stall you because you are eating fat instead of burning the fat you readily have available on your thighs.

If you do not take in enough nutrients, your body will go into starvation mode. If your body goes into starvation mode, it will hold onto every ounce of food you bring in to save for the famine that has surely arrived. That's how this all worked centuries ago when a food stop was not readily available every thirty feet. Let it be known I am calling out those of you who purposely aim to eat only 900 or 1200 calories on your "healing" ketogenic diet. There is nothing healing about taking in less nutrients than a normal person needs just to get out of bed in the morning. If you do this enough, you will continue down the path of poor health and plus size jeans.

There are many people who cannot reach ketosis if they are not taking in enough fat. Their abused bodies refuse to let go of any excess stored fat because they feel deprived of nutrients. These abused bodies do not know when they will next receive nourishment they require to just to complete the most basic of tasks.

The trick with maximizing a ketogenic diet is to eat enough fat to feel satisfied, but not stuffed. You also want to be sure you are digesting that fat properly and it is the high quality types of fat meant for a healing diet, like coconut oil, butter and red meat. Those are saturated fats, the "deadly fats" we have been warned about for decades. I don't know who these people are that are flatlining from overconsumption of coconut oil. The majority of my nutrient intake each day comes from saturated fats. I've never been healthier.

That entire rant was just to say, please quit stomping your metabolism into the ground by obsessively controlling your calories. Stop trying to bring Weight Watchers into a ketogenic diet. They are polar opposites and bringing them together might cause the world to implode. Connect with how you feel, not with how many calories your smartphone shows you have left to consume today.

There I go teaching again when I said this was going to be about cooking tips. Let's get back to cooking tips for lazy gourmet sauces & sides, shall we?

Lazy Gourmet Sauces

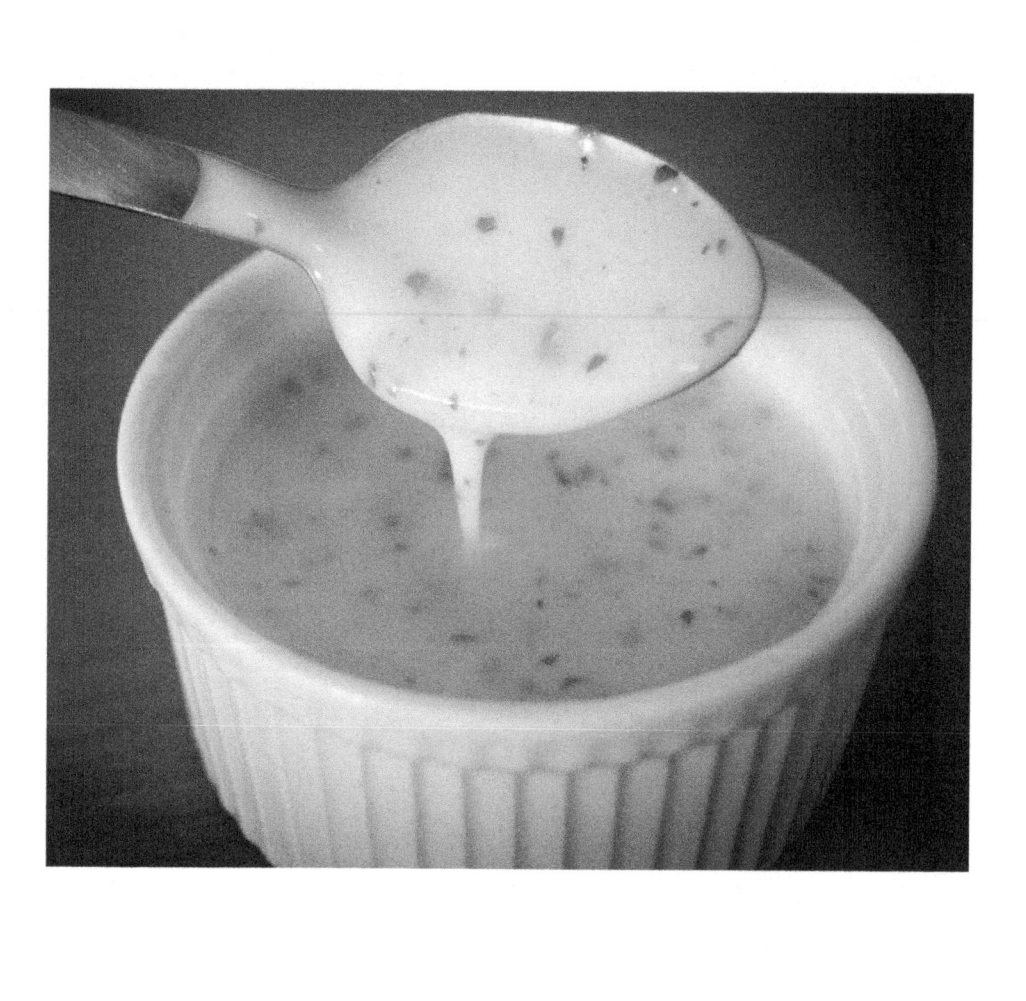

Sauces

You'll notice several recipes throughout the cookbook that use the sauces listed in this section. Please do not feel limited to these recipes. I love to whip up extra of all of the sauces and store them in the fridge to pour over different meal options throughout the week.

My husband adores the creamy garlic sauce almost more than he adores me. He will beg for extra just to pour over eggs and lunch leftovers during the week. The creamy garlic sauce to my husband is equivalent to leftovers for new dinner casseroles to my mother - he will use it on everything!

Don't be concerned regarding the consistency of the creamy garlic sauce or creamy garlic pesto sauce after they are refrigerated. They tend to harden, but they blend together once you heat them up over the stove.

While we are chatting about the stove, time for another quick teaching rant. Please do not use the microwave to reheat any of the recipes found in this cookbook. Yes this is *The Lazy Keto Gourmet*, but using the microwave is taking the lazy factor too far! It is just as easy to use a skillet on the stove. I typically melt a pat of butter first for most leftovers to add flavor and to avoid any meat from sticking.

Using the microwave not only makes the leftovers taste bad, but some people say it even changes the composition of your food. This means your body may no longer recognize it as real food. This can make your real food meal harder to digest.

Creamy Garlic Pesto Sauce

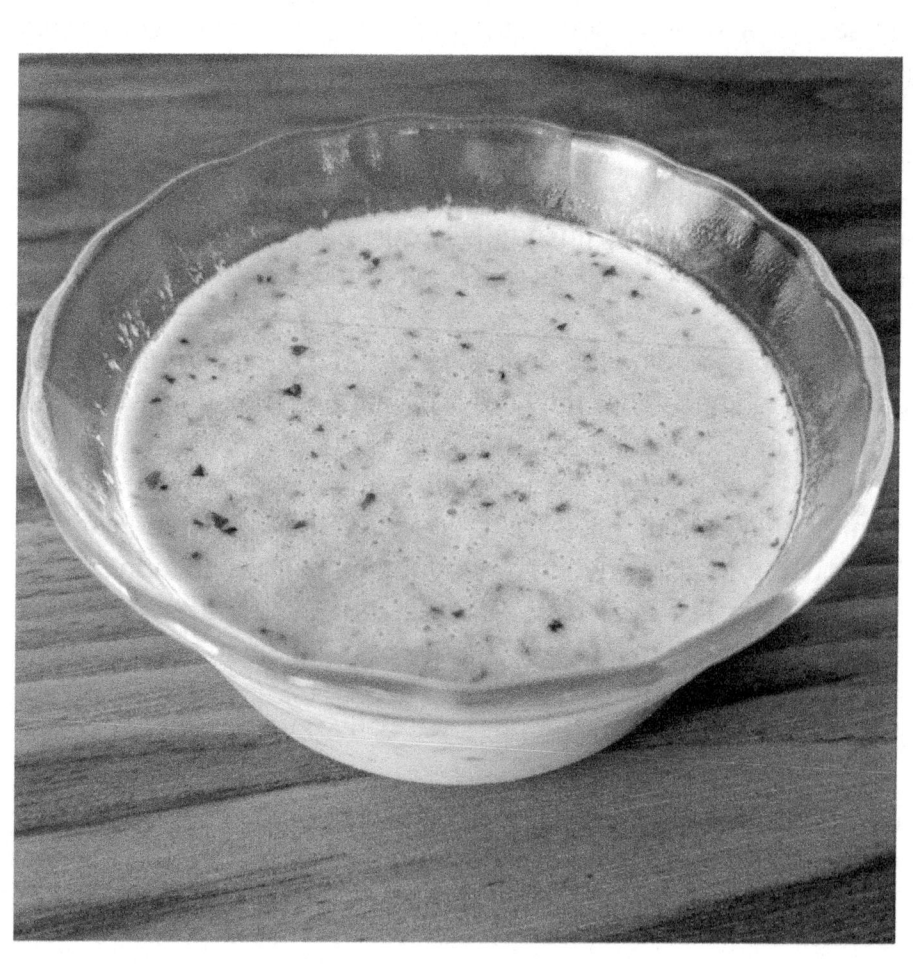

Ingredients:

- ⅓ cup pesto
- ⅓ cup water
- ⅔ cup heavy whipping cream
- 2 tablespoons butter
- 1 teaspoon minced garlic

Directions:

- Heat water and heavy cream in small saucepan over medium heat until hot, but not boiling.
- Stir butter, pesto sauce and minced garlic into saucepan. Whisk ingredients together.
- Reduce heat and cook over low heat for 5 minutes, or until sauce thickens to desired consistency.

Tip: I pour this sauce over easy scrambled eggs to make a high-fat & delicious breakfast that will satiate and energize for hours! This is also great over chicken or seafood.

Garlic Cream Sauce

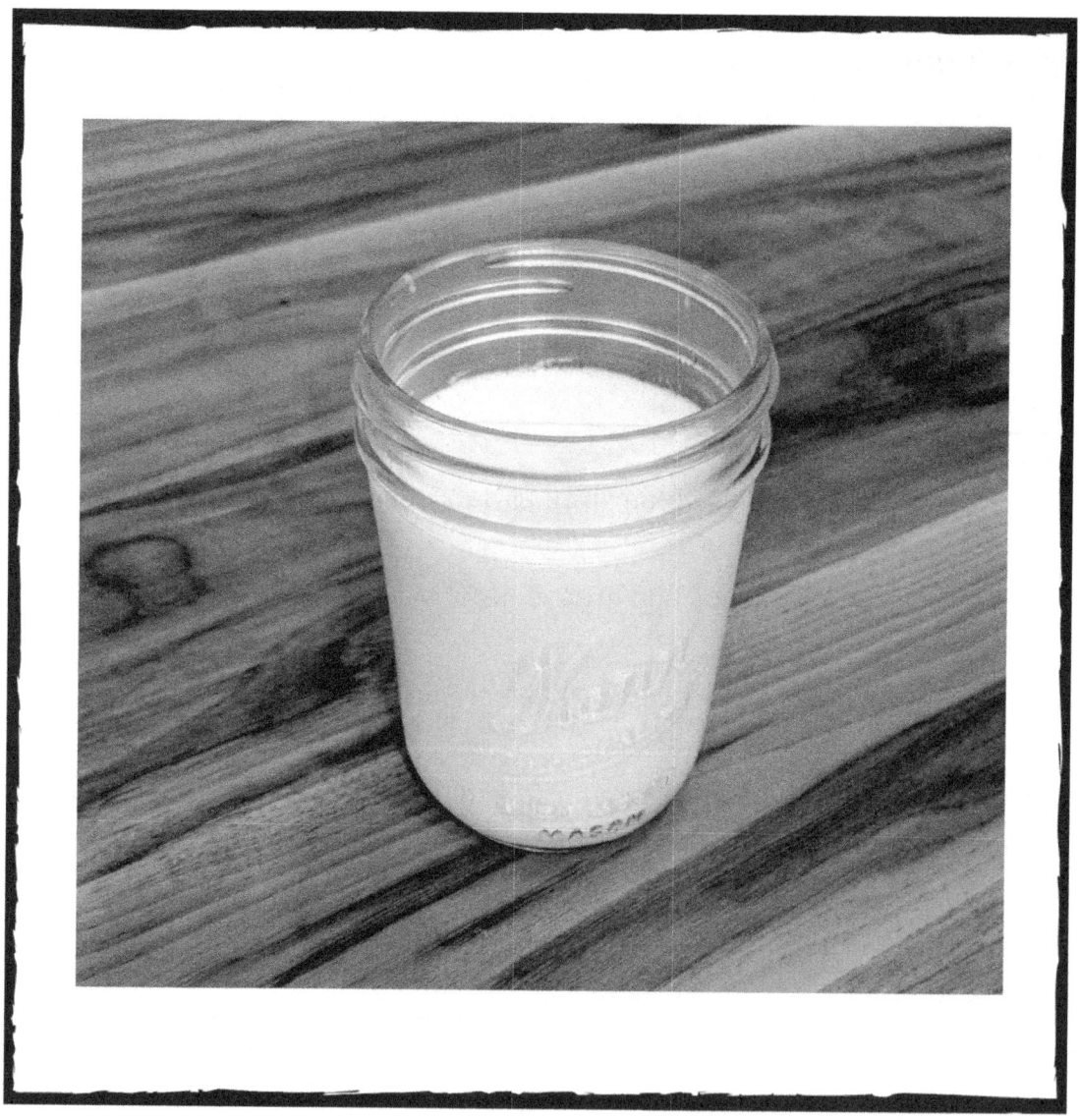

Ingredients:

- 2 cups heavy whipping cream
- 2 teaspoons minced garlic
- 2 tablespoons butter

Directions:

- Melt butter in saucepan.
- Once melted, stir in minced garlic. Cook until lightly browned, or 2-3 minutes.
- Begin to add heavy cream in ½ cup increments.
- Once sauce thickens to desired consistency, add ½ cup cream until all sauce has been added to saucepan and thickened. Total time takes approximately 20 minutes.

Tip: Store leftover sauce in fridge to reheat and pour over chicken, eggs or other leftovers throughout the week.

Bruschetta

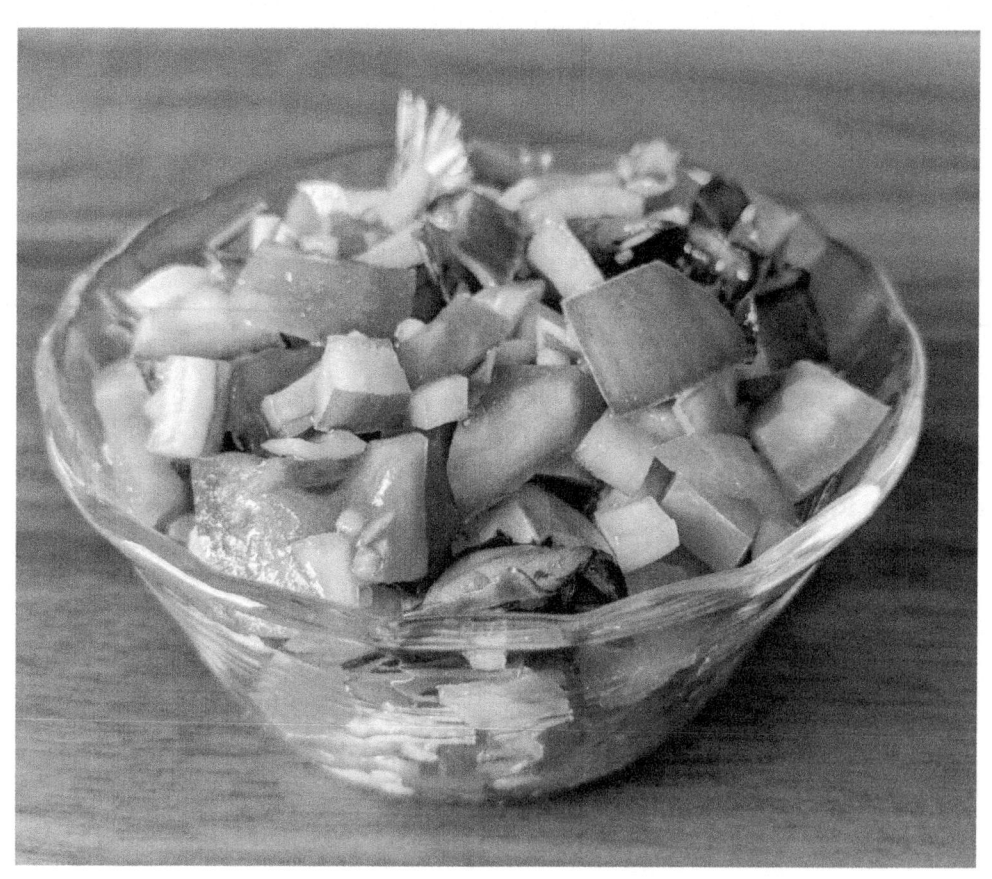

Ingredients:

- 1 large plum tomato, diced
- 1 medium red onion, diced
- 5 leaves fresh basil, chopped
- 1-2 teaspoons minced garlic
- 2 tablespoons olive oil

Directions:

- Combine all ingredients in bowl. Stir well.
- Cover and refrigerate until ready to serve.

TIP: This goes well over chicken or eggs.

Garlic Herb Butter

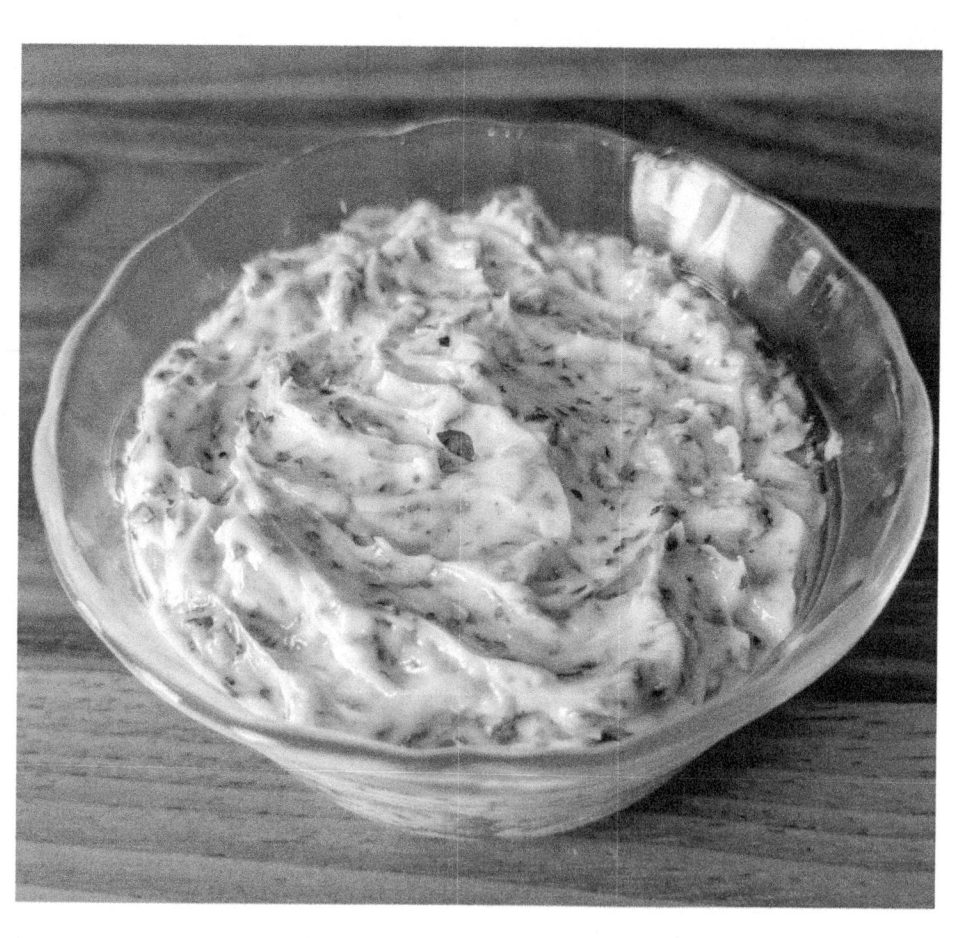

Ingredients:

- 8 tablespoons butter, softened
- 1 tablespoon basil
- 1 tablespoon oregano
- 1 tablespoon chives
- 1 teaspoon minced garlic
- 1 teaspoon parsley
- ½ teaspoon black pepper

Directions:

- Add all ingredients to mixing bowl.
- Beat on low with hand mixer until butter is fluffy.
- Store covered in fridge.

TIP: If you use fresh herbs, the butter will taste fresher, but not last as long. I use dried spices for garlic herb butter that stays fresh longer.

Lazy Gourmet Sides

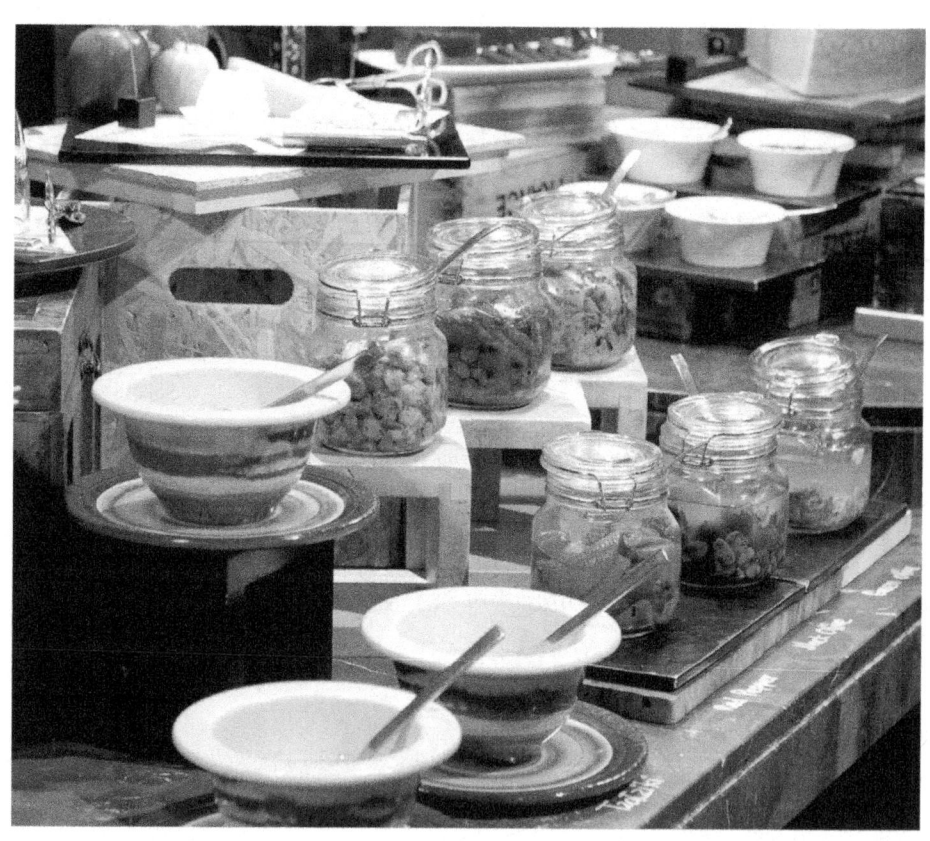

Sides

I list the keto rings first because those are my favorite! I have gone out to fancy steak restaurants before and left sad after I realized this is a side I make and not readily available to order. It should be! These onion rings are delicious. Making them makes a mess, but it is completely worth the cleanup effort.

When you are ready to make the keto rings, really be ready. Clear the kitchen of all the chaos. Here's looking at you jumpy toddlers and husband always standing in the way. You need to move fast to make sure the onion rings do not burn.

When I take the rings out of the fridge, I mix them with my hands once more to make sure they are heavily coated with the egg mixture. I spread the spice mix on a cookie sheet and lay the coated rings over the mix, then flip. Then I throw them into the really hot oil. Do this quickly because once you fill the pan, it will most likely be time to flip the batch. Do not do it so quickly that you splatter the hot oil and burn yourself, because ouch.

If I have a large batch, I will have two large pans filled with very hot oil ready to go. I noticed making a second batch in the same pan tends to burn the onion rings unless you add a lot of oil to the pan. You will also have to scrape away spices in between batches.

Follow the same guidelines for the keto zucchini. You do not have to flip quite as quickly, but don't let it burn. Burnt zucchini is not gourmet.

Regarding the recipes for cauliflower rice: do not tell me you do not like cauliflower if you have not tried any of these recipes. I didn't think I liked it either. Then I made the coconut cauliflower fried rice and fell in love!

The amazing thing about cauliflower is it can be used in place of potatoes or rice in all kinds of sides. It is low carb and makes a great replacement. It somehow counts as a vegetable, even though you wouldn't know it by how awesome it tastes in these recipes.

It can also be found already riced in many stores. Since you are reading a book with lazy in the title, you probably like the sound of that! I like to buy my cauliflower rice at Costco since I go through it very quickly. They also sell an organic version, which makes my body happy.

Keto Rings

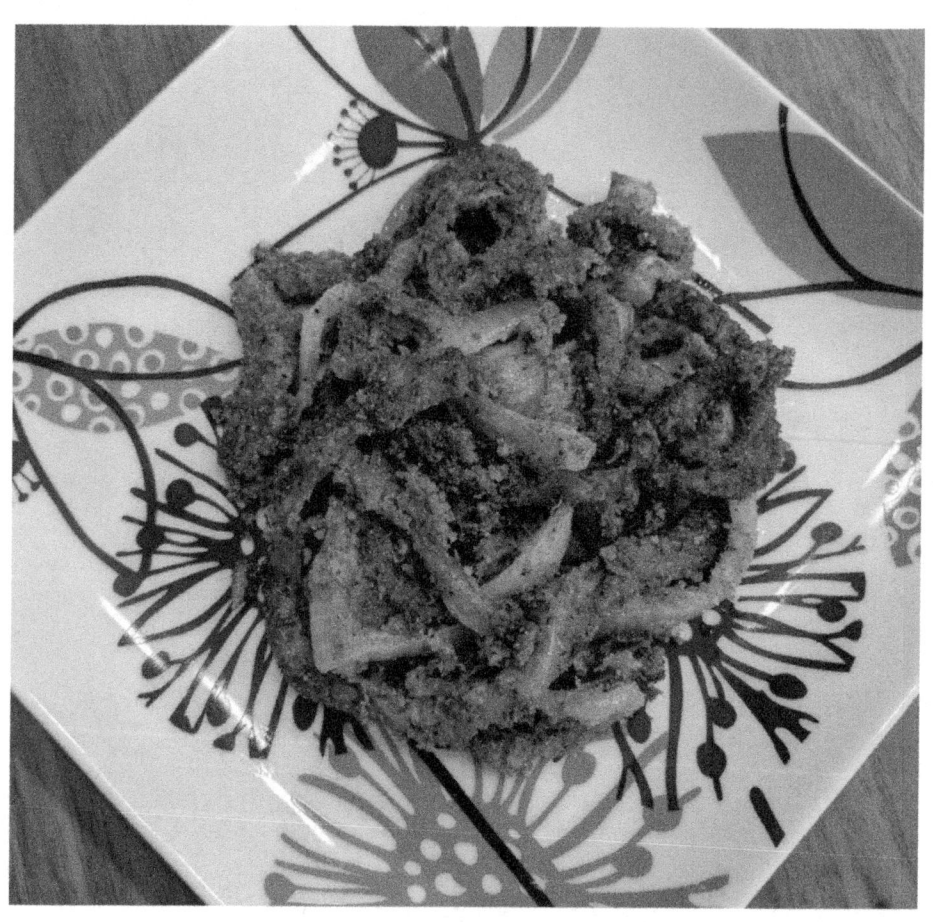

Ingredients:

- 1 large sweet onion
- 1 large egg
- 1 tablespoon heavy whipping cream
- 2 tablespoons coconut flour
- 1 tablespoon baking powder
- ½ tablespoon paprika
- 1 teaspoon garlic powder
- ½ teaspoon salt
- ½ teaspoon black pepper
- ½ teaspoon onion powder
- 2-3 tablespoons coconut oil for frying, or enough to coat bottom of pan once melted

Directions:

- Slice onions into ⅔ inch rings.
- Beat heavy cream and egg together in bowl.
- Pour egg mixture over onions and soak in fridge for 30 minutes.
- Mix coconut flour, baking powder, paprika, salt, pepper, onion powder and garlic powder in mixing bowl.
- Heat coconut oil in large skillet on high heat.
- Pour spice mix onto baking sheet. Flatten with hands into thin layer.
- Remove onions from egg mixture and lay on top of spice mixture. Flip rings to coat both sides.
- Place onions directly into hot coconut oil and fry 1-2 minutes per side.
- Prepare to flip onions quickly so they do not burn.

Fried Keto Zucchini

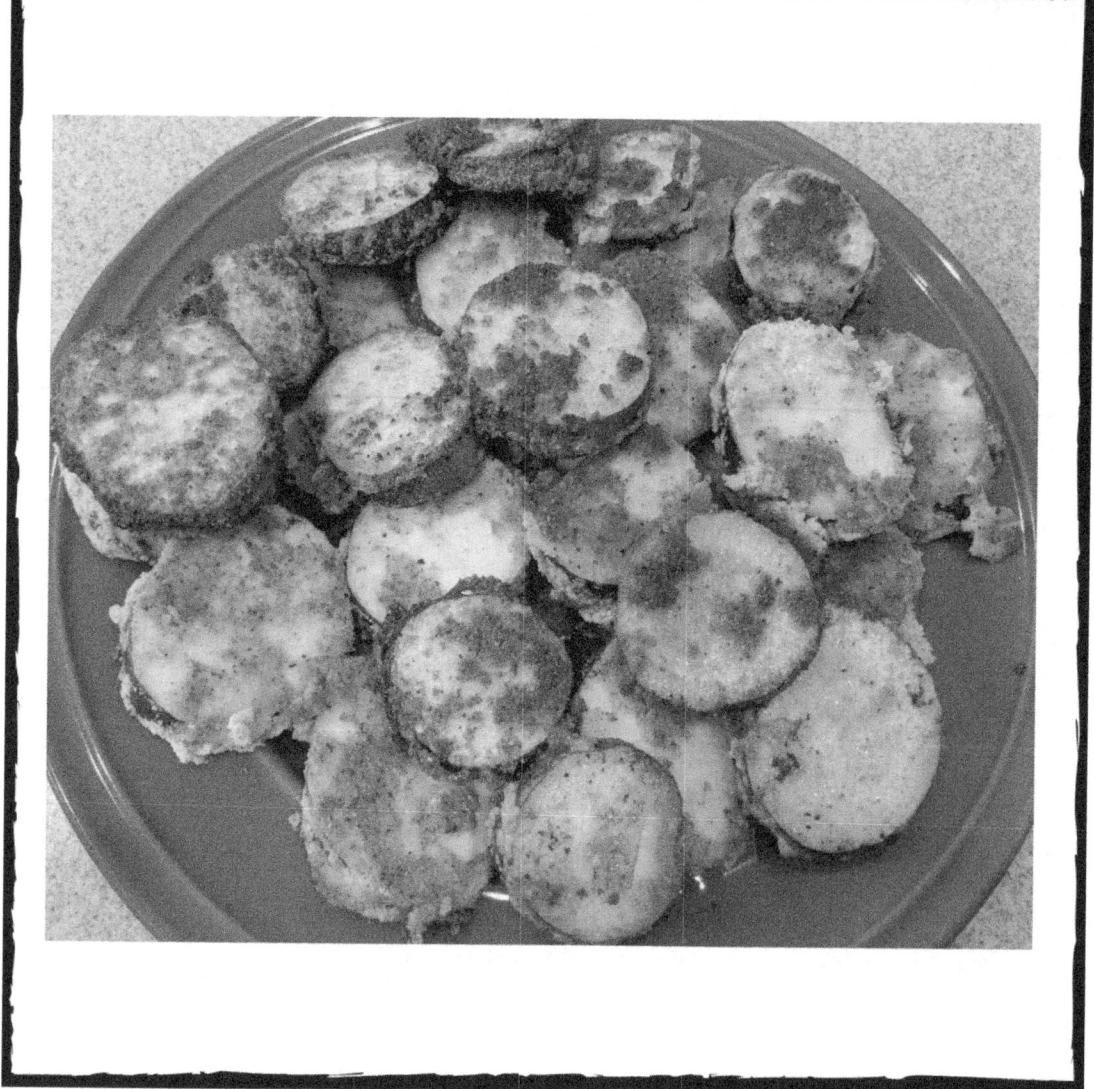

Ingredients:

- 1 large zucchini
- 1 large egg
- 1 tablespoon heavy whipping cream
- 2 tablespoons coconut flour
- 1 tablespoon baking powder
- ½ tablespoon paprika
- 1 teaspoon garlic powder
- ½ teaspoon salt
- ½ teaspoon black pepper
- ½ teaspoon onion powder
- 2-3 tablespoons coconut oil for frying, or enough to coat bottom of pan once melted

Directions:

- Slice zucchini into ½ inch slices.
- Beat heavy cream and egg together in bowl.
- Pour egg mixture over zucchini and soak in fridge for 30 minutes.
- Mix coconut flour, baking powder, paprika, salt, pepper, onion powder and garlic powder in separate shallow bowl.
- Heat coconut oil in large shallow skillet on high heat.
- Pour spice mix onto baking sheet. Flatten with hands into thin layer.
- Remove zucchini from egg mixture and lay on top of spice mixture. Flip zucchini to coat both sides.
- Place zucchini directly into hot coconut oil and fry 1-2 minutes per side.
- Prepare to flip zucchini quickly so they do not burn.

Coconut Sauteed Onions

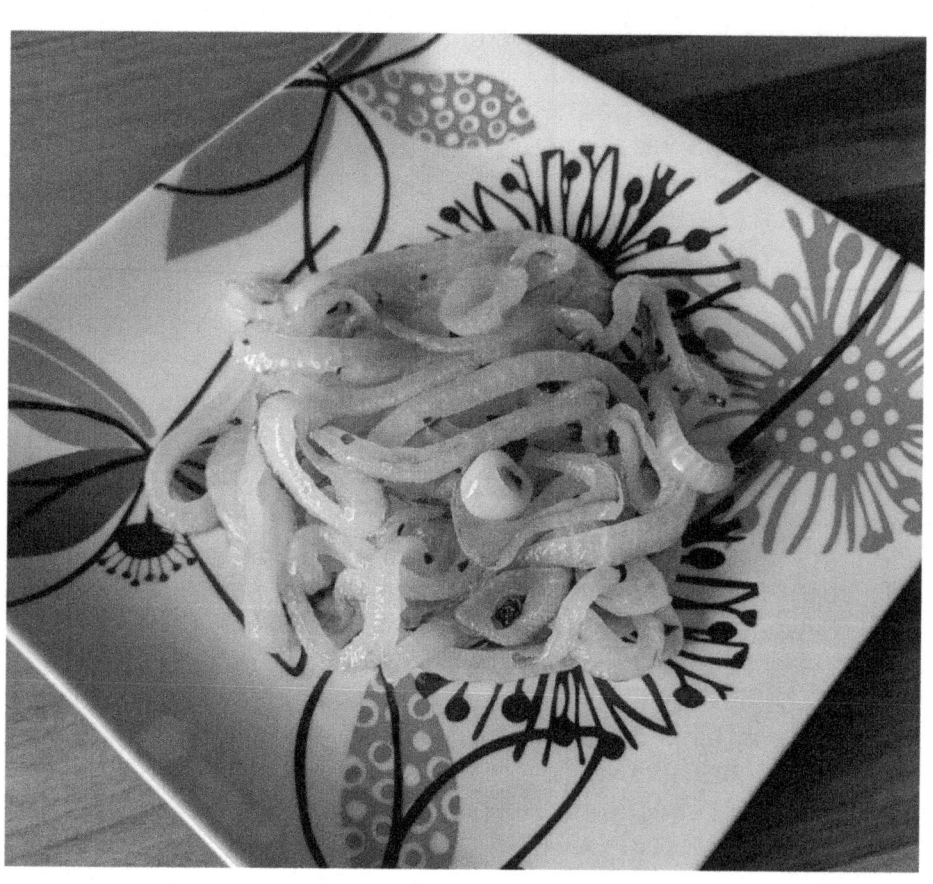

Ingredients:

- 1 large sweet onion
- 2-3 tablespoons coconut oil, or enough to cover bottom of skillet once melted
- 2 teaspoons minced garlic

Directions:

- Slice onion into ½ inch slices.
- Heat coconut oil in large skillet on high heat.
- Once coconut oil is very hot, add onions.
- Stir while cooking.
- After 2-3 minutes, add minced garlic.
- Cook until onions are lightly golden brown.

*Tip: These onions are a great side for hamburgers or grilled sausages.

Creamy Garlic Green Beans

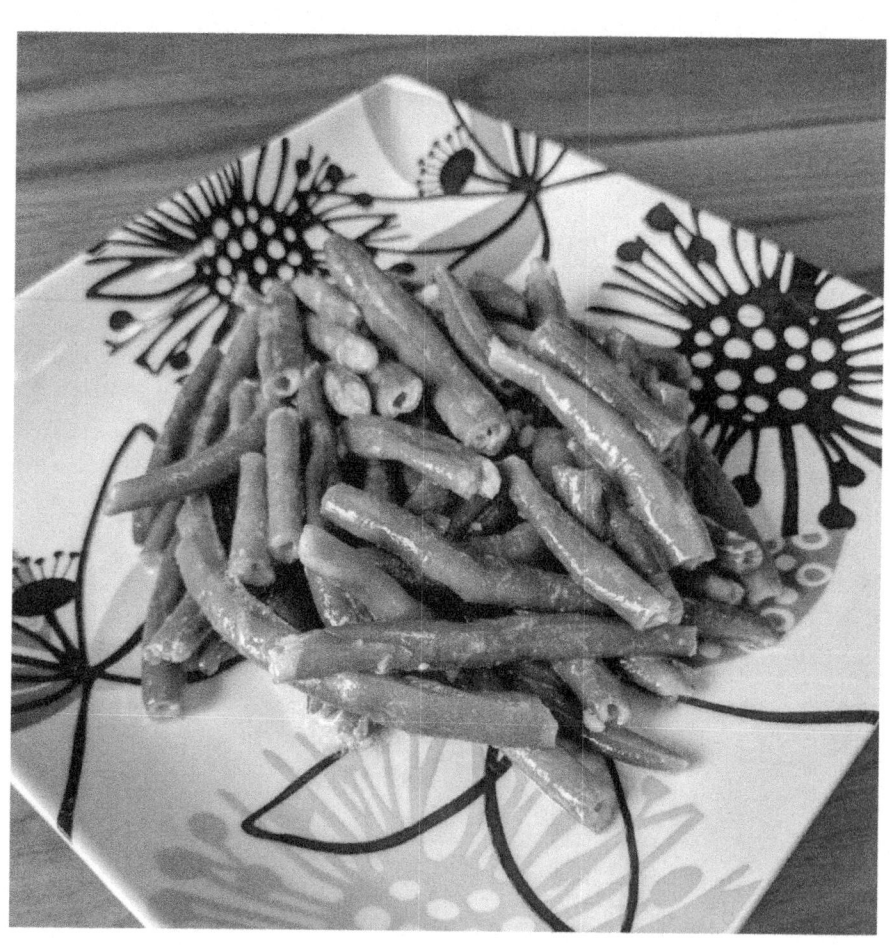

Ingredients:

- 12 ounces frozen green beans
- 4 tablespoons butter
- ¼ cup heavy cream
- 1 teaspoon minced garlic
- Sea salt

Directions:

- Melt butter in saucepan on medium heat.
- Add minced garlic and cook 2-3 minutes.
- Stir in heavy cream.
- Add green beans to saucepan. Bring cream mixture to a boil.
- Turn heat to medium, cover and cook for 5-10 minutes, or until sauce thickens and green beans are cooked. Stir occasionally while cooking.
- Season with sea salt.

Coconut Cauliflower Fried Rice

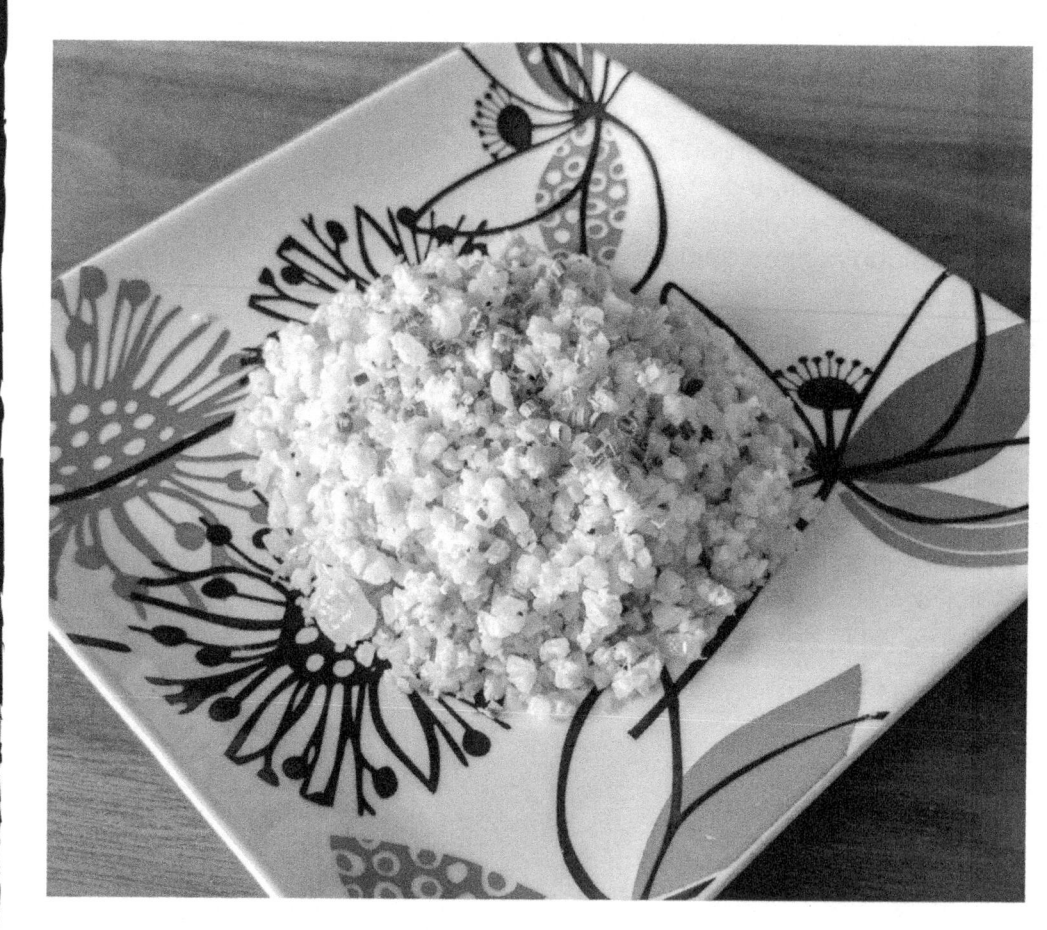

Ingredients:

- 1 bag riced cauliflower. Alternatively, you can rice your own. In this instance, use 1 medium head of cauliflower.
- 1 large egg, beaten
- 2-3 tablespoons coconut oil, or enough to cover bottom of skillet when melted
- ½ medium sweet onion, chopped
- 2 green onions, diced
- 2 teaspoons minced garlic
- 2 tablespoons coconut aminos
- Black pepper
- Sea salt
- If you prefer vegetable fried rice, additional chopped vegetables to consider: celery, broccoli, green or red peppers, spinach

Directions:

- In large skillet, melt coconut oil over medium-high heat.
- Once melted, add onion and minced garlic. Cook 2-3 minutes, or until onion has softened.
- Add riced cauliflower. Cook until tender but not mushy, approximately 5 minutes.
- Mix in coconut aminos and black pepper. Stir.
- Pour egg slowly over rice to coat most of rice. Stir well until egg is fully cooked.
- Remove from heat. Stir in diced green onions and sea salt.

Garlic & Herb Cauliflower Rice

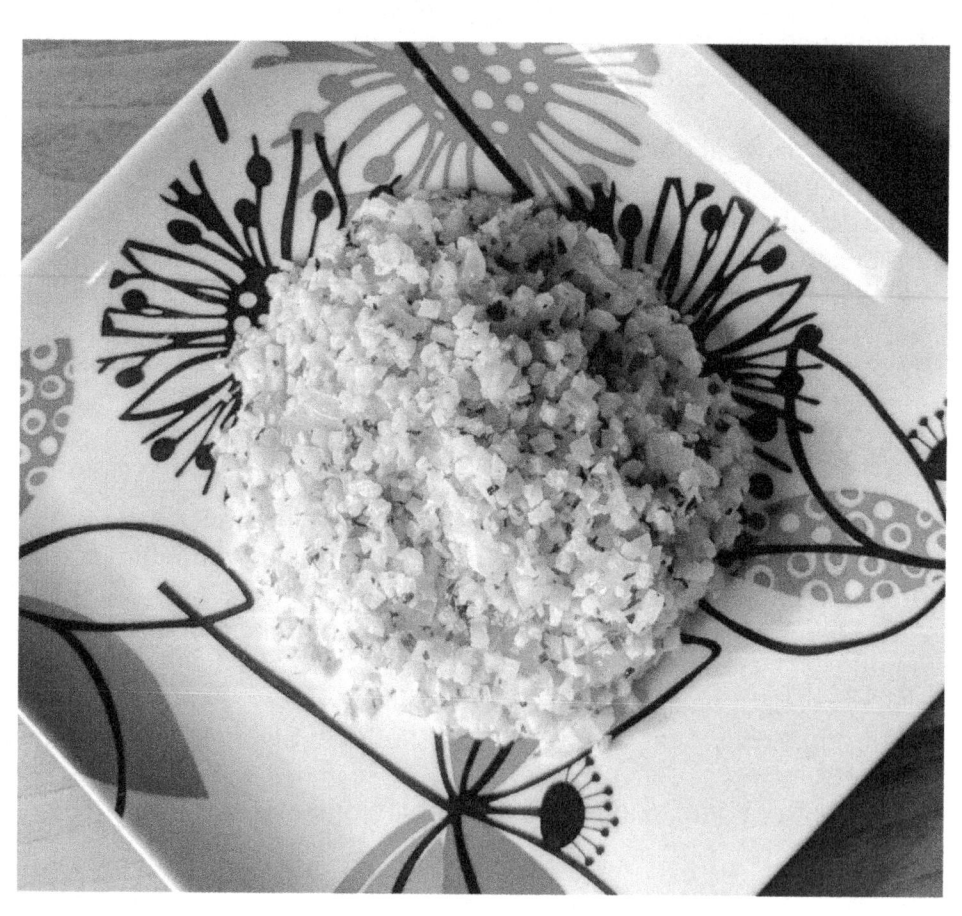

Ingredients:

- 1 bag riced cauliflower
- 4 tablespoons garlic herb butter
- 1 small sweet onion, diced
- 1 teaspoon minced garlic
- Sea Salt
- Black pepper

Directions:

- Melt 2 tablespoons garlic herb butter in large skillet on low heat.
- Once melted, add diced onion and minced garlic. Cook over medium heat for 2-3 minutes, or until onions soften.
- Add riced cauliflower. Cook until tender but not mushy, approximately 5 minutes. Stir while cooking.
- Add additional garlic herb butter. Cook until butter melts and rice is cooked fully.
- Season to taste with salt and pepper.

Mexi-Caulirice

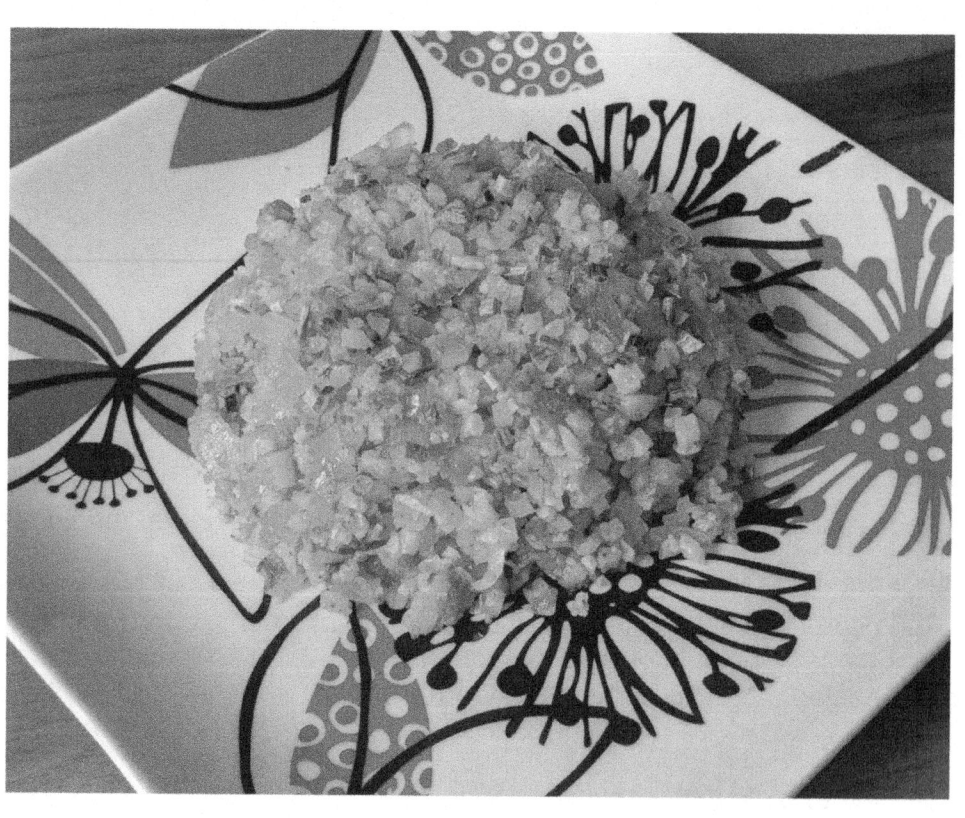

Ingredients:

- 1 bag riced cauliflower
- 2-3 tablespoons coconut oil, or enough to cover bottom of skillet when melted
- 1 small sweet onion, diced
- 2 teaspoons minced garlic
- ½ teaspoon ground cumin
- ½ teaspoon chili powder
- ½ teaspoon sea salt
- ¼ teaspoon oregano
- ¼ teaspoon cayenne pepper
- 3 tablespoons fresh salsa
- Green onions, chopped

Directions:

- Melt coconut oil in skillet on medium heat.
- Once melted, add diced onion and minced garlic. Cook for 2-3 minutes, or until onions soften.
- Add riced cauliflower. Cook until tender but not mushy, approximately 5 minutes. Stir while cooking.
- Season with cumin, chili powder, sea salt, oregano and cayenne pepper. Stir well.
- Remove from heat. Stir in salsa.
- Garnish with chopped green onions.

Cheesy Cauliflower Rice

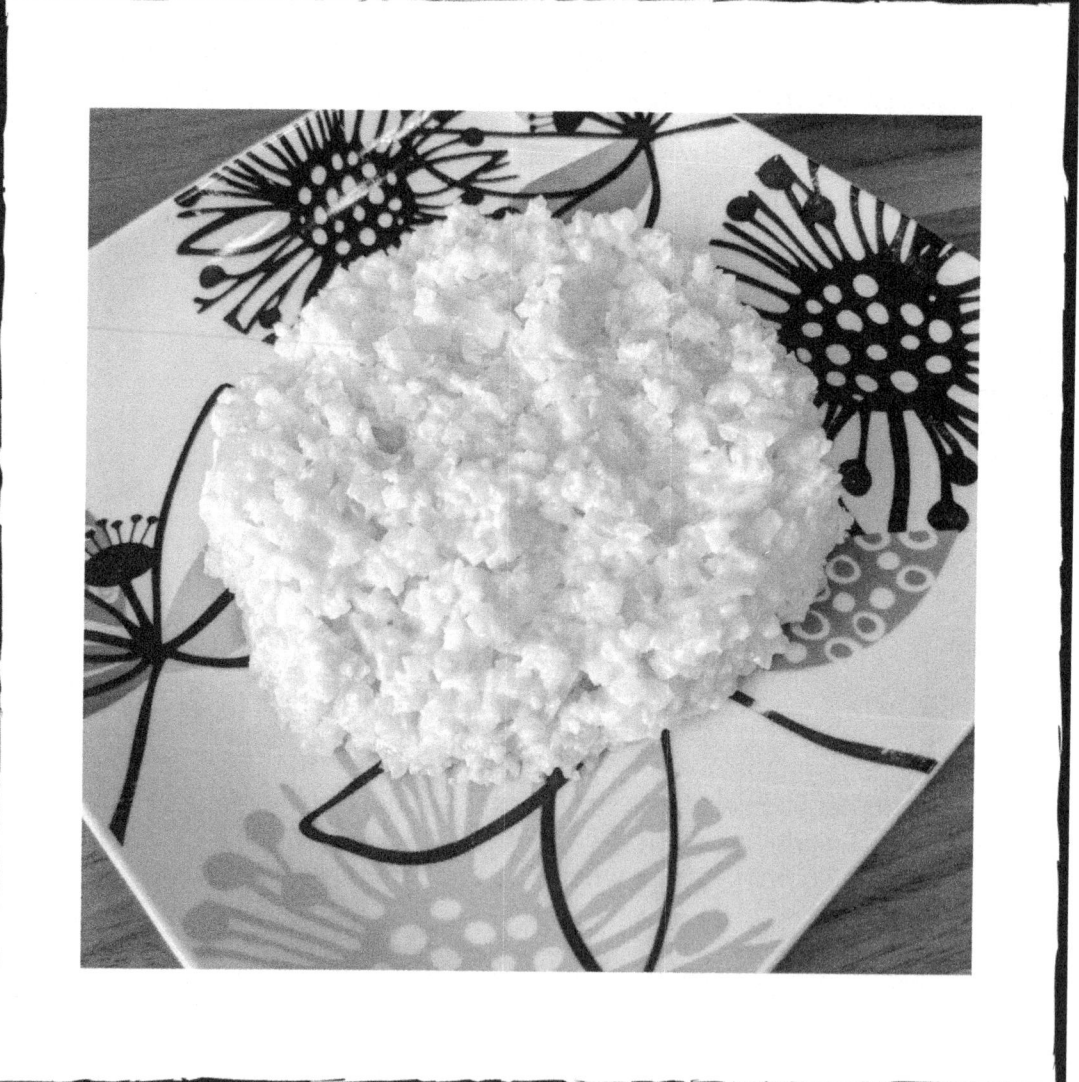

Ingredients:

- 1 bag cauliflower rice
- 2 tablespoons butter
- 1 cup finely chopped onion
- 2 teaspoons minced garlic
- 8 tablespoons full fat cream cheese
- 3 tablespoons heavy cream
- ½ teaspoon onion powder
- Sea salt
- Black pepper

Directions:

- Melt butter over low heat in a large skillet.
- Stir in onions and minced garlic. Cook over medium heat for 2-3 minutes, or until onions soften.
- Stir in riced cauliflower. Cook until tender but not mushy, approximately 5 - 10 minutes. Stir as you cook.
- Reduce heat to low.
- Stir in cream cheese, heavy cream and onion powder. Season with salt and pepper to taste.
- Stir over low heat until cheese is melted, or approximately 2 minutes.

Lazy Gourmet

Fat Bombs

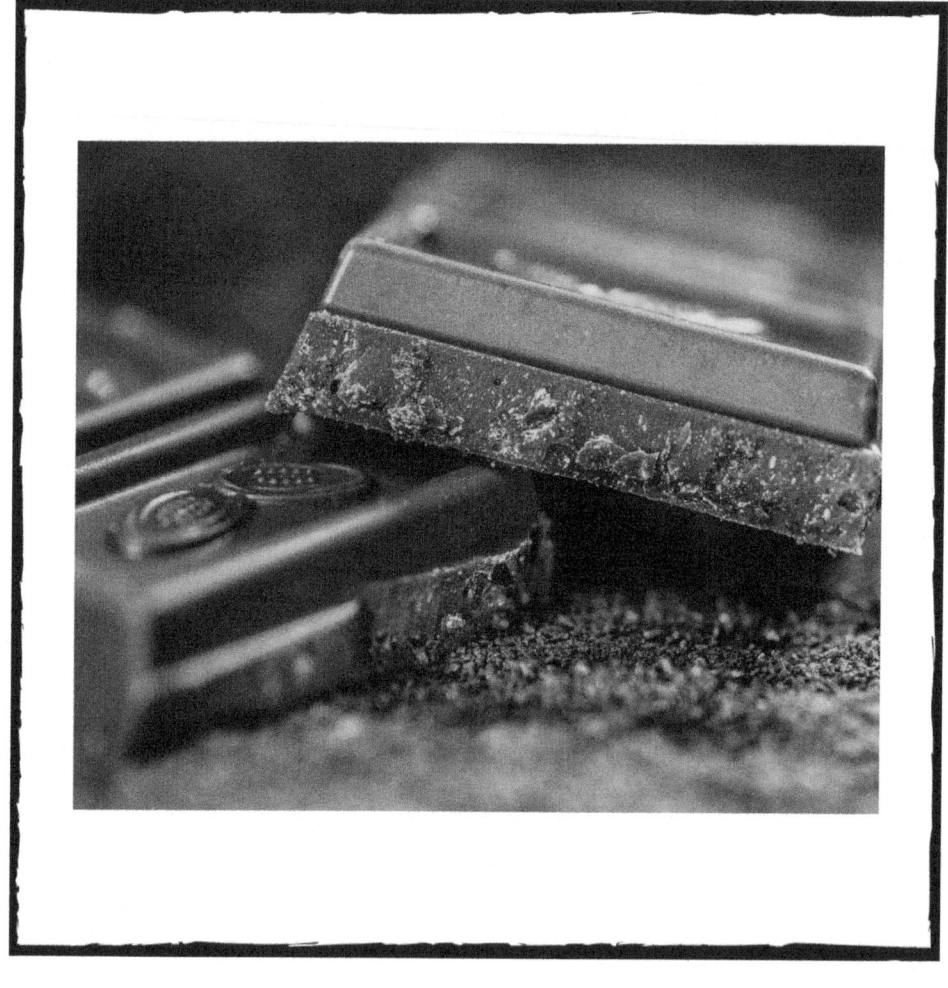

Fat Bombs

Perhaps you've heard of fat bombs before, but do not understand the purpose they serve. Fat bombs are kind of my jam, so we are about to do some learning up in here.

The first fat bomb I ever made is called a coconut yummy. This is a recipe from *Kick Your Fat in the Nuts*. TC explains to use fat bombs like this as a trick to help your body learn how to efficiently burn fat as fuel. If you are wondering who the heck TC is, he is the author of *Kick Your Fat in the Nuts*. We are on a first name basis because I am kind of a teacher's pet.

This logic goes back to the point I explained before: if you do not have enough fat coming in, your body will be reluctant to let go of stored fat on your body. This is a fact of life no matter how many people scream at you that you need to take in less fat in order to burn the fat on your body. Perhaps and maybe this is more true once your body becomes fat adapted. You will never become fat adapted if you are limiting the amount of fat you take in at the start of your ketogenic diet. When you are at the beginning, you need to eat all the fat!

TC further explains you want to consume these fat bombs after your meal. The reasoning behind this is fat is going to be hard to digest for most people. As a nation we have been told for years the evils of fat, so a lot of us stopped eating it. This means our bodies forgot what to do with fat and views healthy fats as a toxic invader. Your body is now going to fight back against this toxic invader in the form of diarrhea, acne, itchy skin and the like. One way to help with this is by adding Beet Flow to your routine. You already learned all about this in the digestion course.

To my knowledge you can only get Beet Flow from Natural Reference. Beet greens you find in health stores is not the same thing. If you choose to purchase Beet Flow from Natural Reference, I ask that you use my Practitioner Code at checkout: nissahelpsme. Also, email me for instructions so you are using the supplements correctly.

Another way to help your body learn to digest fat is to consume it at the end of the meal. Your body's digestive functions are already in full motion, so adding fat at the end will help. If you are not digesting fats well, ramping your intake up slowly will also help. I understand some proponents of the ketogenic diet scream, "Let's eat all the fat!' They are wrong.

Wait a minute….didn't I just get done telling you to eat all the fat?

Yes, yes I did. In order to lose stored body fat you need to take in adequate amounts of healthy fats. If you are not digesting those fats properly, it doesn't matter how much healthy fat you take in. You are going to store some of it as toxins (excess fat) and spitfire rage the rest out of your backside. We talked about this already, remember?

If you are experiencing the digestive symptoms that come along with too much fat, you need to perform a balancing act while working on digesting your fats better. Take in enough to feel good, but not too much where you get sick. This will be different for everyone, so you have to put in the work to figure this out for yourself. Increase your intake overtime as you feel ready.

Another thought about fat bombs. Some of my favorite teachers say fat bombs are unnecessary on a ketogenic diet. They tout a ketogenic diet is all about the real food and sweet treats like fat bombs are just fueling our desire for evil sugary treats of the past.

I disagree. I put my money where my mouth is because some days half of my diet is made up of fat bombs. This only makes me crave more healthy fats, not sugary cupcakes.

Most of the fat bombs I make are made up mostly of coconut oil or butter. Those are the real foods we are supposed to be eating on a ketogenic diet. I would prefer not to eat a pat of butter or spoonful of coconut oil by itself when I need extra fat. When I mix butter or coconut oil with dark chocolate, now we are talking!

Part of the debate regarding fat bombs is all of the added artificial sweeteners. I too previously added too many artificial sweeteners to fat bombs. The sweeteners have zero calories; what's the harm? Turns out, a lot of harm.

Too many artificial sweeteners, even the "natural" kinds like stevia and Swerve, can cause cravings, rises in insulin and harm to gut bacteria. All of these side effects mean more fat around your waist. I wrote an entire blog about artificial sweeteners in case you want to learn more.

I gave up artificial sweeteners in January 2018. All forms of stevia and Swerve were out of my diet for more than six months before I performed an experiment. I added a few drops of liquid stevia to my coffee. BIG MISTAKE. I felt weak, I felt shaky and my body thought it hadn't eaten in 40 days and 40 nights. I also had a pounding headache for three days following my experiment.

When you bombard your body with things it does not take well to daily, you might not notice the side effects. When you eliminate possible harmful foods for at least a month or two and then try to reintroduce them one at a time, it is easier to detect if these foods are right for you. Artificial sweeteners clearly are not right for me. I did not realize this prior to removing them completely. I will not make that mistake again.

This brings up an important point to the recipes in this cookbook that is worth repeating. I do not use artificial sweeteners in any of the recipes. If you currently live on sweetened foods, artificial or otherwise, some of these recipes are going to be too bitter for you. Add sweeteners at your own risk. My suggestion is to wean yourself down until you do not require any unnecessary sweeteners in your food. After going unsweetened for a while, you won't miss the fake stuff. I didn't believe it at first either.

I now consume my fair share of fairtrade 85% dark chocolate, but that is as sweet as I get. My body no longer craves excess sugar or carbs because I took away the fake sweetness that was causing the cravings in the first place. My gut health is also improving one day at a time without the unnecessary sweeteners in my food. This is a big deal, even if you still don't believe me.

Peanut Butter Bombs

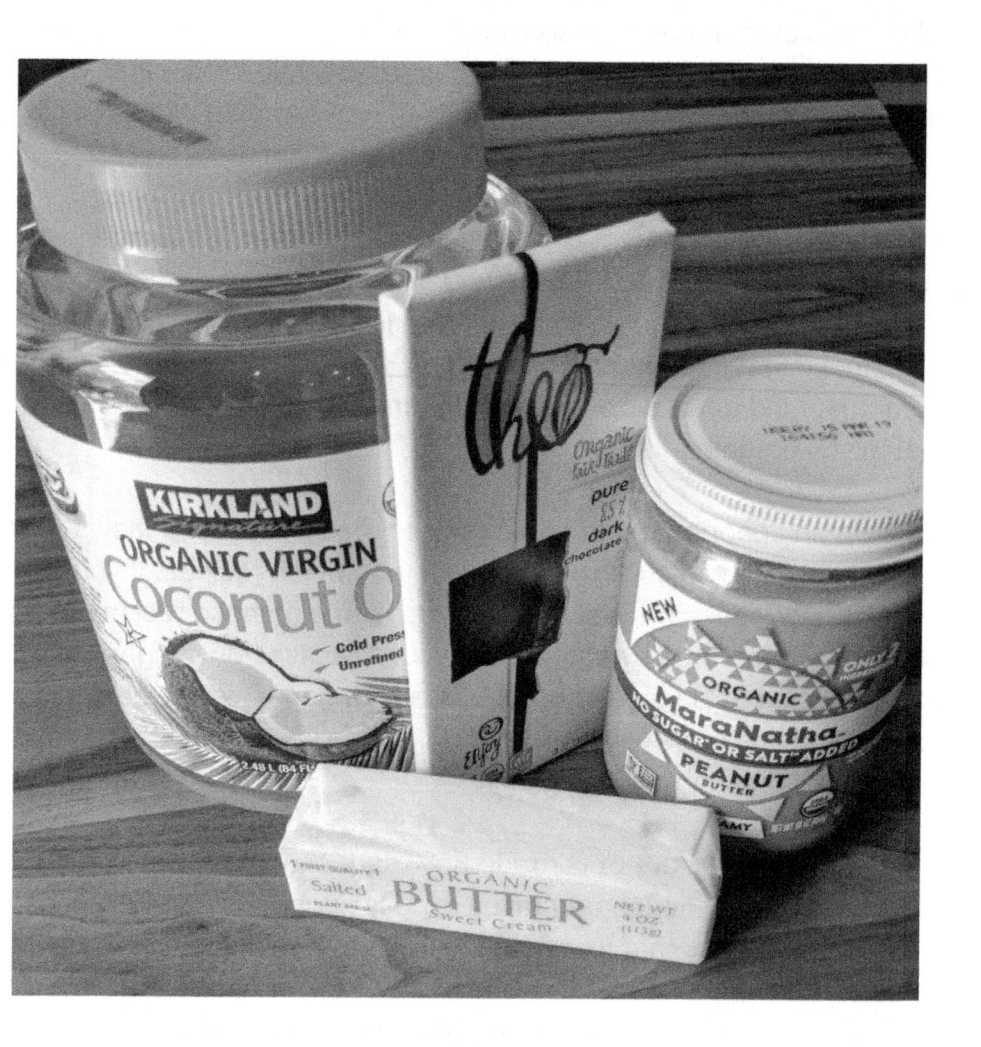

Ingredients:

- 8 tablespoons coconut oil
- 4 tablespoons butter
- 4 tablespoons peanut butter
- 1 ounce dark chocolate

Directions:

- Combine coconut oil, peanut butter, butter and dark chocolate into medium saucepan. Melt ingredients over low heat.
- Stir with whisk occasionally while melting.
- Spoon into mini muffin pan in 1 tablespoon increments.
- Freeze until firm, approximately 20 minutes.
- Remove from pan by popping out with butter knife.
- Store in ziploc bag in freezer or fridge.

* Recipe makes approximately 24 fat bombs

Chocolate Almond Butter Bombs

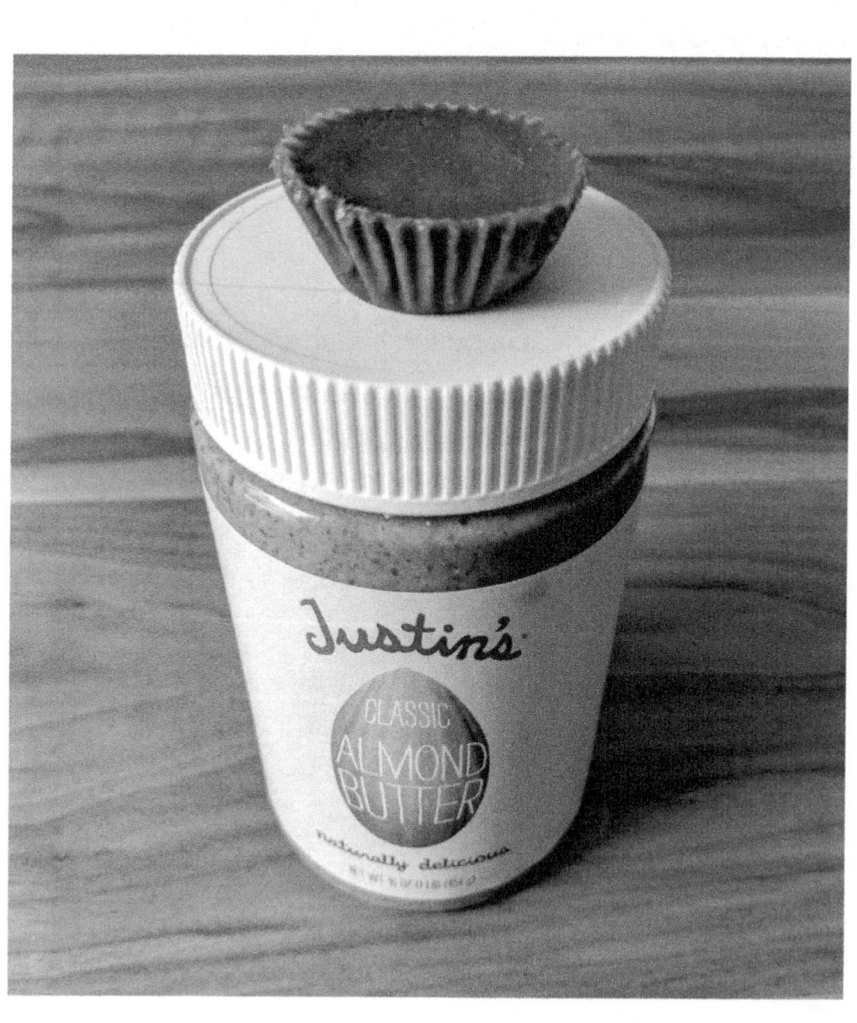

Ingredients:

- 8 tablespoons almond butter
- 8 tablespoons coconut oil
- 2 ounces dark chocolate
- 3 tablespoons heavy whipping cream, room temp.
- ⅛ teaspoon vanilla extract

Directions:

- Layer mini muffin pan with liners.
- In saucepan, combine almond butter, dark chocolate and coconut oil. Melt ingredients over low heat.
- Stir with whisk occasionally while melting.
- Remove from heat and allow to cool for 2-3 minutes.
- Stir in heavy cream and vanilla extract. Whisk all ingredients until smooth.
- Pour mixture into tins in 1 tablespoon increments.
- Place in freezer until firm, approximately 20 minutes.
- Store in ziploc bag in fridge or freezer.

*Makes approximately 24 fat bombs

Minty Melts

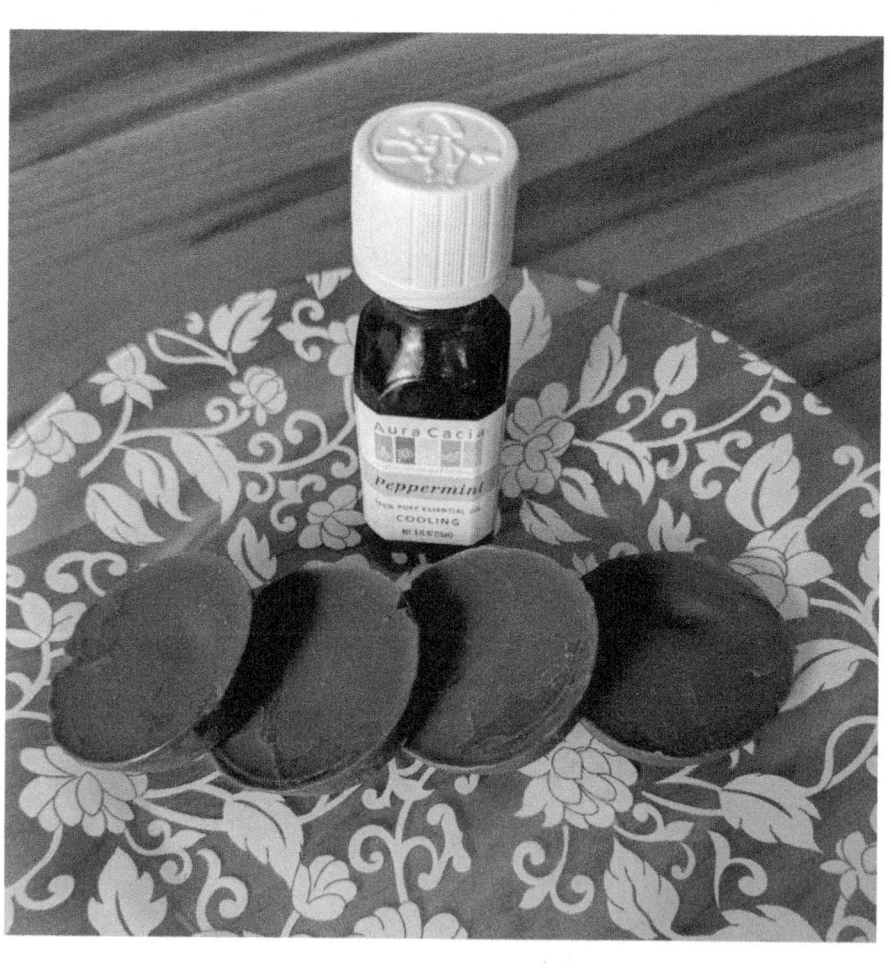

Ingredients:

- 10 tablespoons coconut oil
- 4 ounces dark chocolate
- ⅛ teaspoon vanilla extract
- 4 drops peppermint essential oil

Directions:

- In medium saucepan, melt dark chocolate and coconut oil over low heat.
- Stir with whisk occasionally while melting.
- Once melted, allow to cool for 2-3 minutes.
- Stir in vanilla extract and peppermint oil.
- Pour into mini muffin pans in 1 tablespoon increments.
- Place in freezer until firm, approximately 20 minutes.
- Pop out of muffin tins with a butter knife.
- Store in fridge or freezer in ziploc bag

Makes approximately 24 fat bombs

TIP: *I double the batch size and store in the freezer. These deliciously melt in your mouth straight from the freezer.*

Caramel Apple Bombs

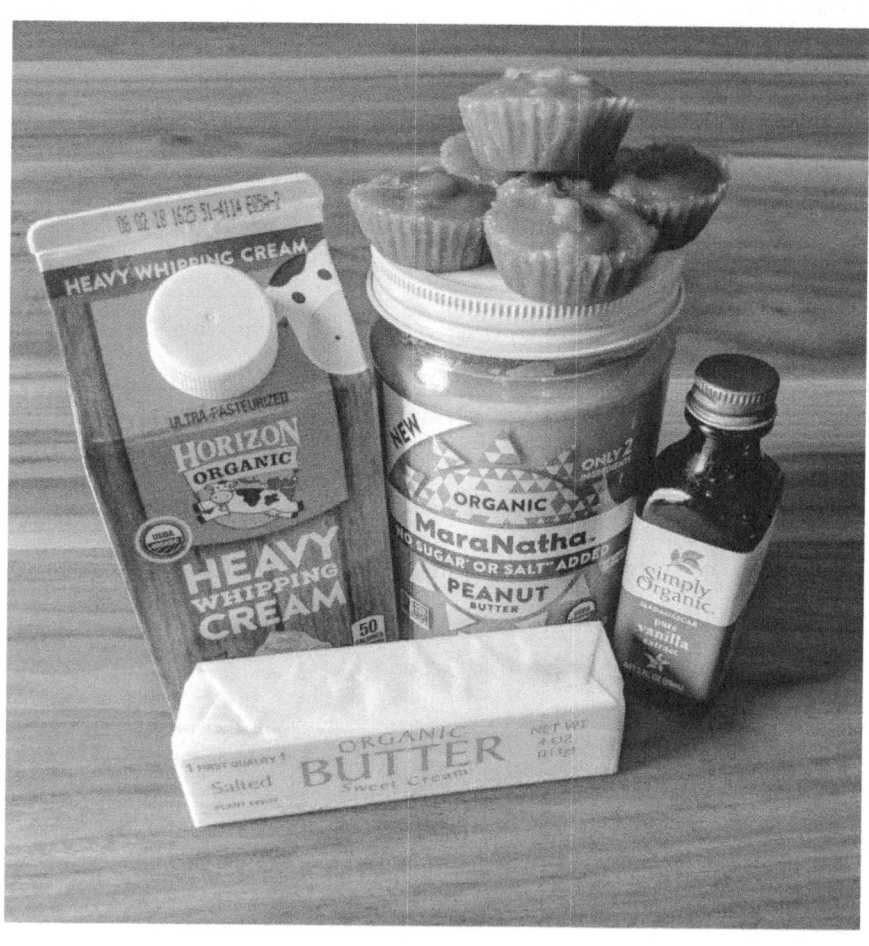

Ingredients:

- 1 cup crunchy no-stir peanut butter
- 8 tablespoons butter
- 4 tablespoons heavy whipping cream
- ⅛ teaspoon vanilla extract

Directions:

- Layer mini muffin pan with liners.
- Melt butter and peanut butter together over low heat in medium saucepan.
- Stir with whisk until well combined.
- Once melted, remove from heat. Allow to cool for 2-3 minutes.
- Whisk in vanilla extract and heavy cream.
- Spoon into mini cupcake liners in 1 tablespoon increments.
- Place in freezer until firm, approximately 20 minutes.
- Remove and store in fridge or freezer in ziploc bag.

*Makes approximately 24 fat bombs

*TIP: There are two ways to enjoy these tasty fat bombs:

- Straight out of the fridge or freezer like a typical fat bomb.
- Melt 1-2 fat bombs in a toaster oven at 350 degrees for 5 -7 minutes for an extra gooey treat (just like the caramel apple topping).

Cheesecake Bombs

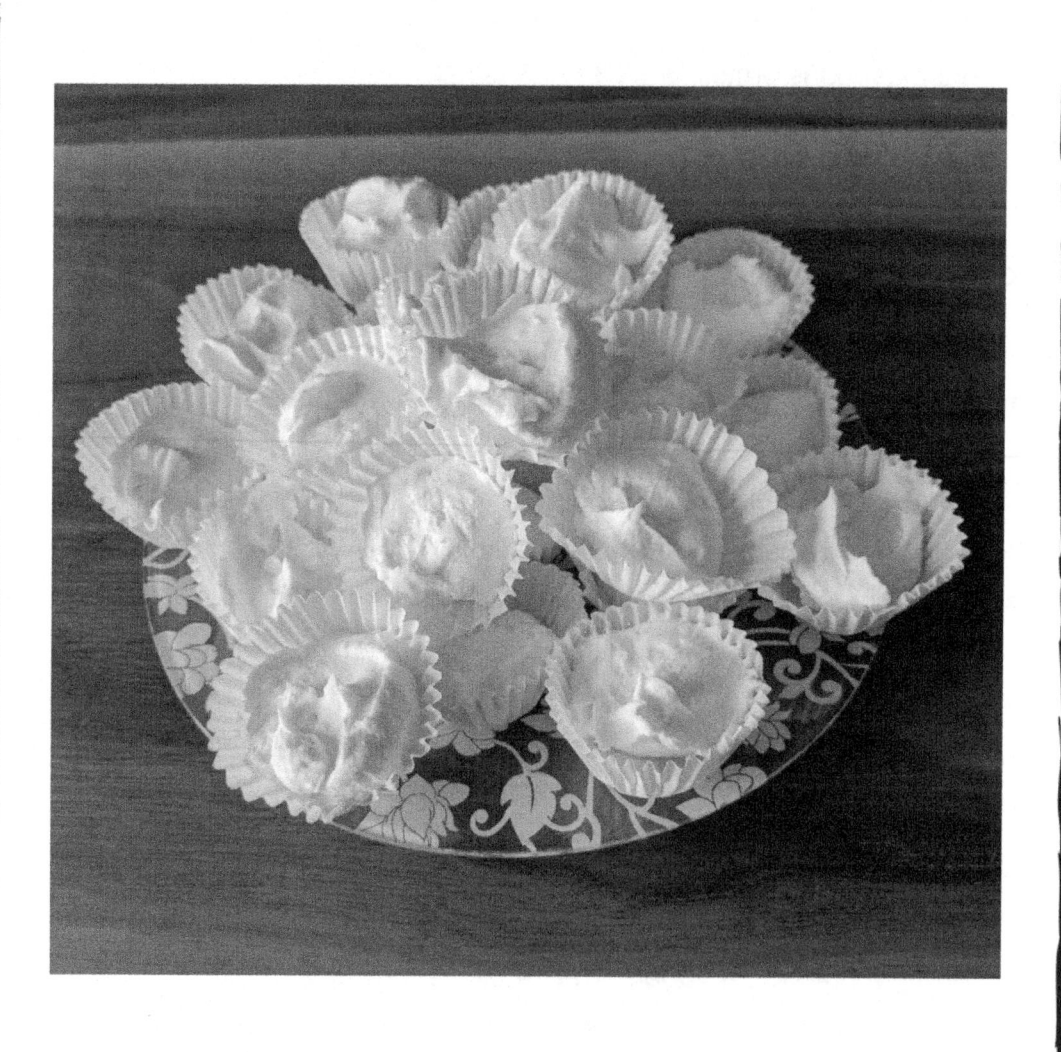

Ingredients:

- 8 ounces cream cheese, softened
- 8 tablespoons butter, softened
- 3 tablespoons coconut oil
- ½ teaspoon vanilla extract

Directions:

- Layer mini muffin pan with liners.
- In large mixing bowl, beat cream cheese until light and fluffy with hand mixer.
- Add butter, vanilla extract and coconut oil. Beat with hand mixer until well combined.
- Spoon into mini cupcake liners in 1 tablespoon increments.
- Place in freezer until firm, approximately 20 minutes.
- Store in ziploc bag in freezer or fridge.

Makes approximately 24 fat bombs

TIP: If cheesecake mixture sticks to hand blender, hold blender over bowl above ingredients and slowly move speed up until mixture is back in bowl.

Chocolate Butter

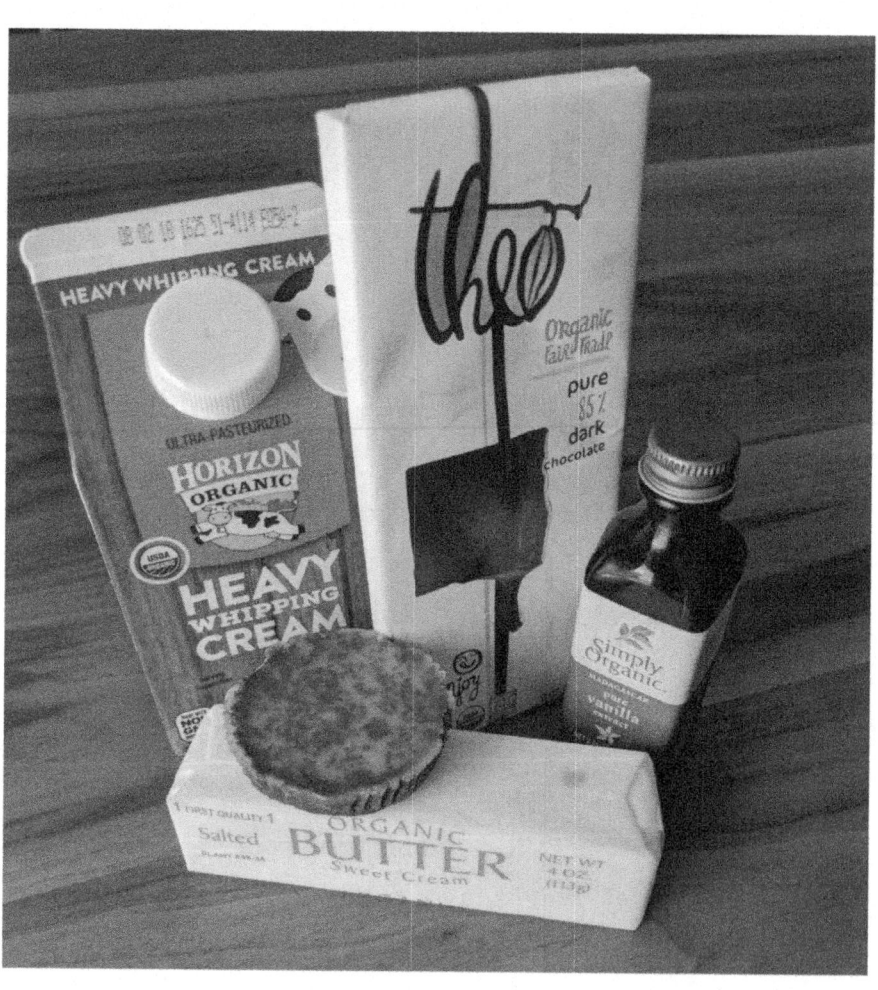

Ingredients:

- 8 tablespoons butter
- 2 ounces dark chocolate
- 3 tablespoons heavy whipping cream, room temp.
- ⅛ teaspoon vanilla extract

Directions:

- Line cupcake tray with cupcake tins.
- Melt chocolate and butter together over low heat.
- Stir with whisk occasionally while melting.
- Once melted, allow to cool for a few minutes to avoid curdling.
- Whisk in heavy cream and vanilla extract. Combine well.
- Add mixture to cupcake tins in 2 tablespoon increments.
- Place in freezer until firm, approximately 20 minutes.
- Place bombs in ziploc bag and store in fridge.

*Makes approximately 8 fat bombs

Walnut Fudge Bombs

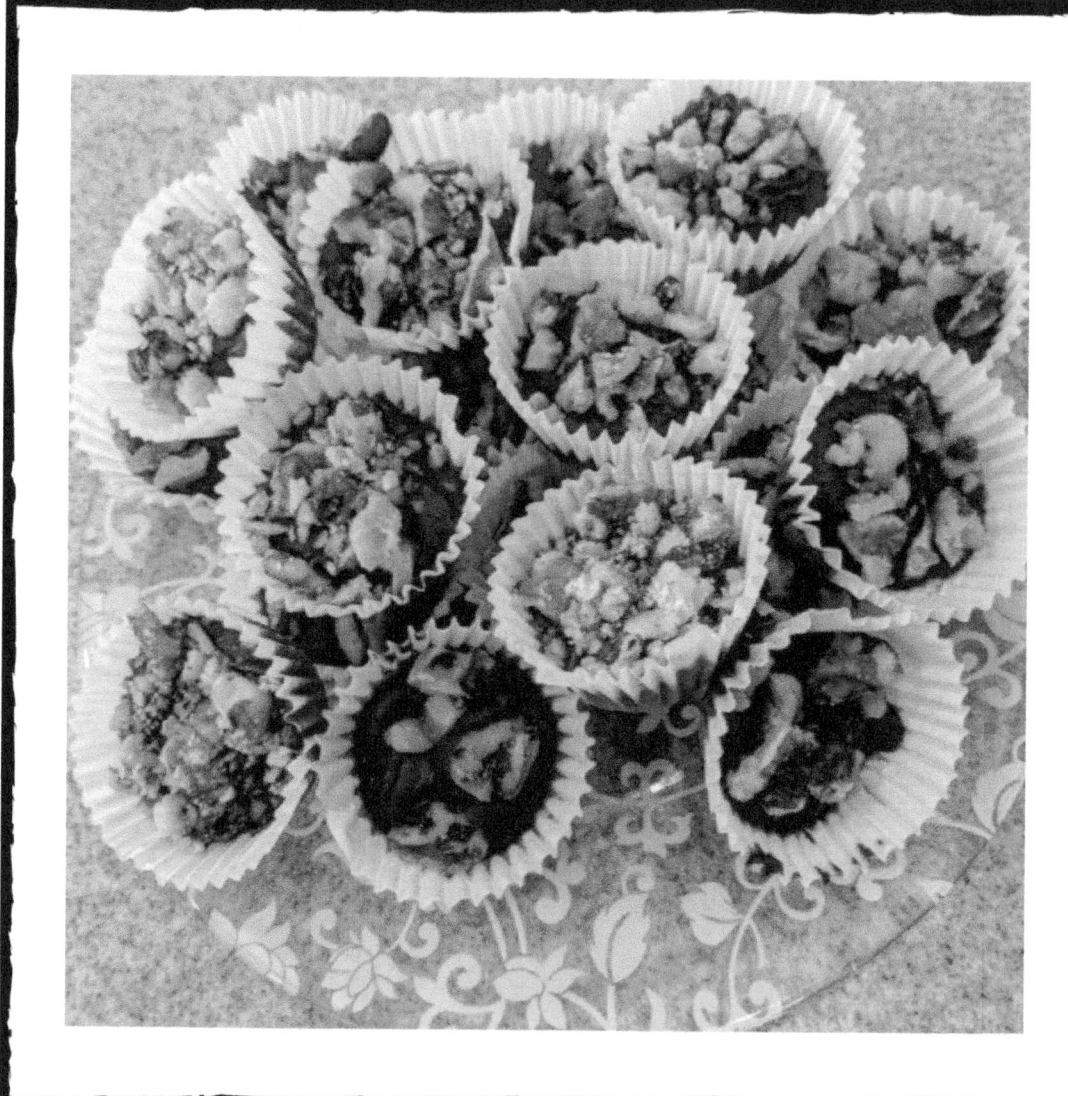

Ingredients:

- 6 ounces dark chocolate
- 8 tablespoons butter
- 6 tablespoons heavy whipping cream, room temp.
- ⅛ teaspoon vanilla extract
- ½ cup walnuts, chopped

Directions:

- Layer mini muffin pan with liners.
- Melt chocolate and butter together over low heat.
- Whisk occasionally while melting.
- Once melted, set aside for a few minutes to cool to avoid curdling.
- Whisk in heavy cream and vanilla extract. Combine well.
- Add mixture to mini muffin tins in 1 tablespoon increments.
- Sprinkle chopped walnuts over fudge bombs.
- Place in freezer until firm, approximately 20 minutes.
- Place bombs in ziploc bag and store in fridge.

*Makes approximately 24 fat bombs

Dark Chocolate
Peanut Butter Cups

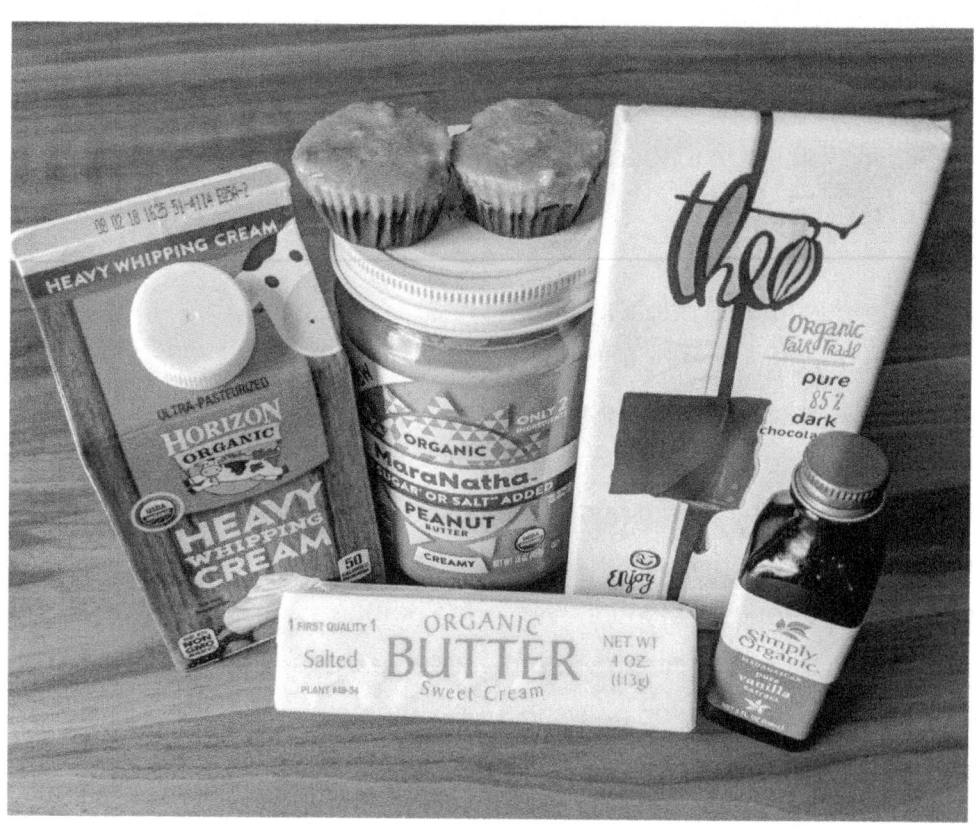

Ingredients:

Chocolate Layer:

- 3 ounces dark chocolate
- 4 tablespoons butter
- 3 tablespoons heavy whipping cream, room temp.
- ⅛ teaspoon vanilla extract

Peanut Butter Layer:

- 3/4 cup peanut butter
- 4 tablespoons butter, melted
- ½ teaspoon vanilla extract

Directions:

- Layer mini muffin pan with liners.
- Melt chocolate and 4 tablespoons butter together over low heat.
- Stir with whisk occasionally while melting.
- Once melted, set aside for a few minutes to cool to avoid curdling.
- Whisk in heavy cream and vanilla extract.
- Add chocolate layer to mini muffin tins in ½ tablespoon increments.
- Place in freezer until first layer is firm, approximately 5-10 minutes.
- Combine peanut butter, melted butter and vanilla extract in mixing bowl.
- Remove muffin tray from freezer. Add peanut butter layer over chocolate layer in ½ tablespoon increments.
- Place in freezer until firm, approximately 20 minutes.
- Place bombs in ziploc bag and store in fridge.

*Makes approximately 24 fat bombs

Maple Pecan Bombs

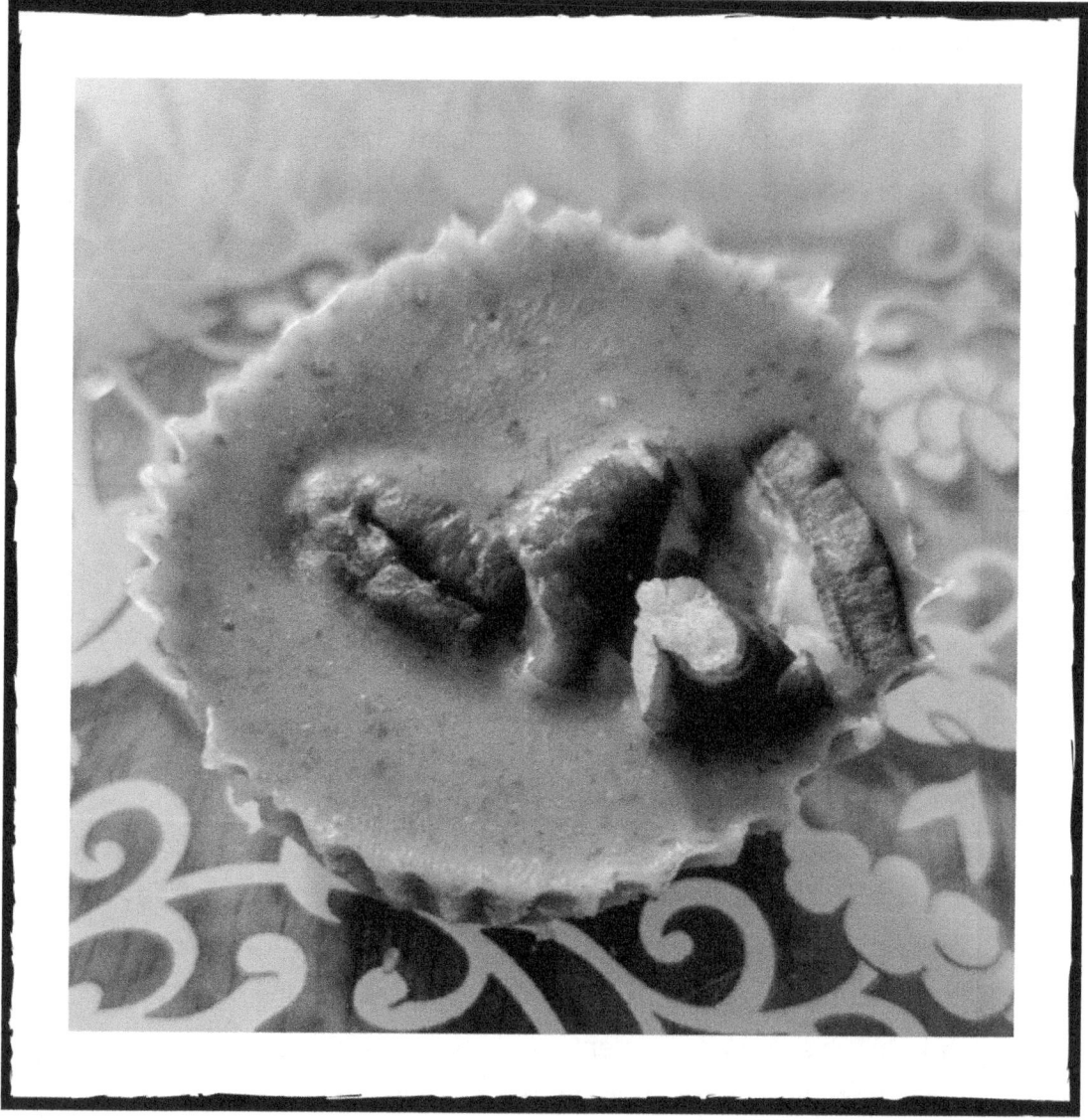

Ingredients:

- 8 tablespoons coconut oil
- 8 tablespoons almond butter
- ¼ cup heavy cream
- 1 teaspoon blackstrap molasses
- ½ teaspoon maple extract
- ⅛ teaspoon vanilla extract
- ¼ cup pecans, chopped

Directions:

- Layer mini muffin pan with liners.
- Melt coconut oil and almond butter in medium saucepan over medium heat.
- Stir occasionally with whisk while melting.
- Once melted, remove from heat and allow to cool for a few minutes.
- Add in heavy cream, vanilla extract, maple extract and blackstrap molasses.
- Stir with whisk to combine.
- Add mixture to mini muffin liners in 1 tablespoon increments.
- Drop in pecans to individual tins by hand.
- Place in freezer until firm, approximately 20 minutes.
- Store in a ziploc bag in fridge or freezer.

*Makes approximately 24 fat bombs

Whipped Cream with Chocolate Butter Sauce

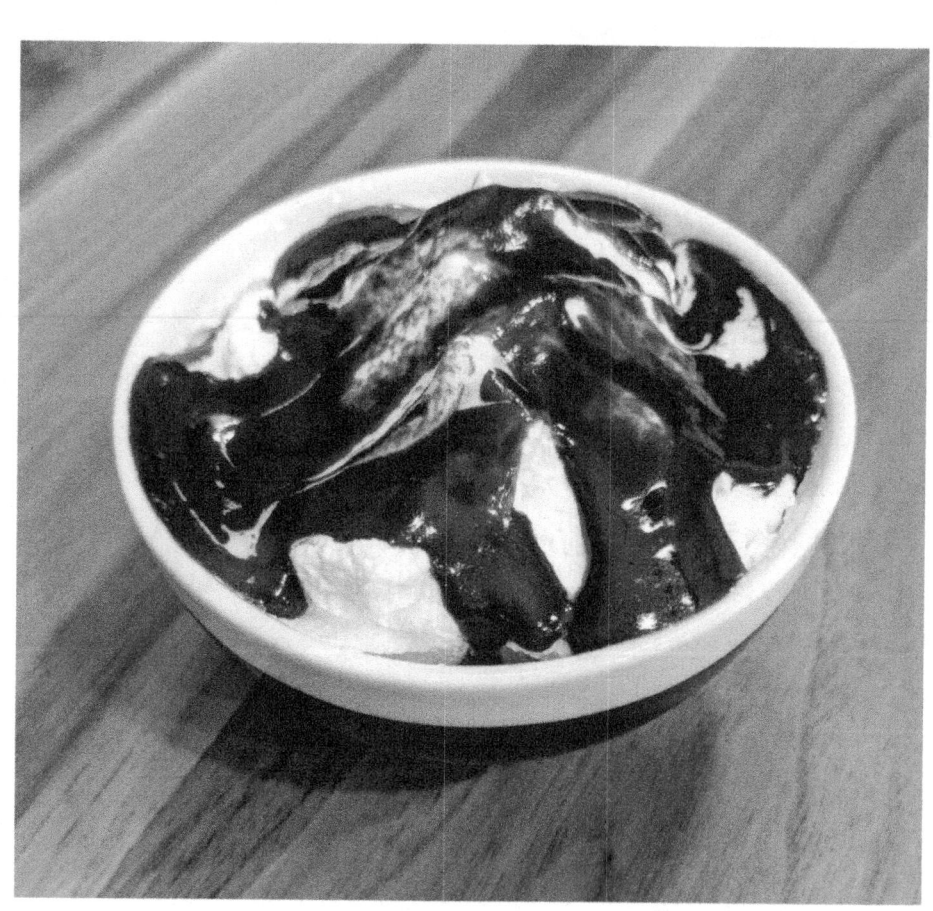

Ingredients:

- 1 cup heavy whipping cream
- ½ teaspoon vanilla extract
- 1 ounce dark chocolate
- 2 tablespoons butter

Directions:

- Melt dark chocolate and butter together over low heat. Stir occasionally.
- Pour heavy cream and vanilla extract into large mixing bowl.
- Beat on high with hand mixer until cream is light and fluffy, approximately 5-10 minutes.
- Drizzle chocolate butter over whipped cream.

Quality Ingredients I Love

As stated earlier in this book, I shop mostly at online marketplaces like Thrive Market to save both time and money. If you click through the affiliate link on my website, you will save 25% off your first order and get free delivery. You will also help me continue my work with Eating Fat is the New Skinny by providing a small affiliate commission, which I do appreciate.

Below is a list of high quality ingredients I currently order from Thrive Market for the recipes listed in this book. Most of them can also be found at local stores, but I find I do save a lot of money ordering through Thrive while also not having to drag two fidgety toddlers in search of ingredients at the store. That is a win in any mom's book!

Items I Order at Thrive Market:

- Emperor's Kitchen Organic Chopped Garlic
- Theo's 85% Dark Chocolate
- Simply Organic Vanilla Extract
- Spectrum Naturals Coconut Spray
- King Arthur Almond Flour
- Justin's Almond Butter
- Bragg Organic Apple Cider Vinegar
- Thrive Market Organic Extra Virgin Olive Oil
- Coconut Secret Organic Coconut Aminos
- Annie's Organic Worcestershire Sauce
- Selina Naturally Celtic Sea Salt
- Simply Organic Basil
- Simply Organic Oregano
- Simply Organic Black Pepper
- Simply Organic Garlic Powder
- Simply Organic Thyme
- Simply Organic Paprika
- Simply Organic Cayenne Pepper
- Simply Organic Ground Cumin

My Daily Menus

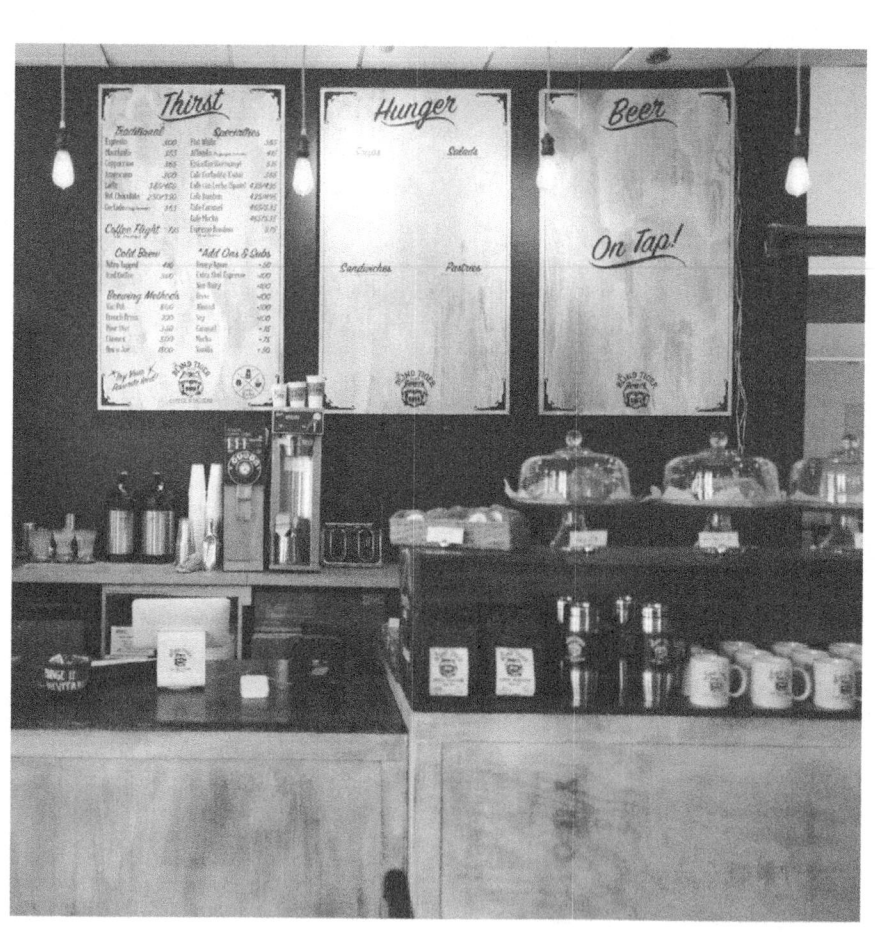

My Daily Menus

The daily menus I consume are going to vary considerably to the menus anyone else reading this cookbook might eat. We are all different people with different body chemistries. You may not love the amount of garlic I eat in a day because maybe you don't want all of the vampires to die with a quick whiff of your breath. Perhaps you like dark chocolate, but do not want to feel like you are lost in *Willy Wonka's Chocolate Factory* by eating dark chocolate with every meal. Maybe your body chemistry requires you to eat more mono or polyunsaturated fats, while mine requires more saturated fats to stay balanced. We all need to take time to figure this out for ourselves.

Obviously you can figure out what you like to eat. That part is easy. If you have no idea what food is ideal for your body chemistry, take the digestion course. Figure it out. Eat the foods that are right for your body chemistry to make this health and weight loss stuff much easier on yourself!

Most people are so used to consuming the SAD diet that when they have to add a bunch of fat to their day, they have no idea where to start. Should they just dip a spoon into a jar of full fat mayo and go for it? Are they supposed to eat a pound of bacon in the morning and another pound for lunch? And what's with all of the people eating pure coconut oil straight from little plastic baggies?

In case you are confused, I am going to provide you with a week's worth of my daily menus. You will see how I personally combine all of these delicious fats together to make up a ketogenic diet that is appropriate for my body. These are the menus I have had success with for losing weight and regaining my health. Keep in mind, my daily menus have changed considerably from where I started. I changed these as my digestion improved and tastes changed. You can copy my week if you would like, but I cannot guarantee the same results. Remember, we are two different people.

Fat

Did you take the time to improve your digestion so your body recognizes fat as an appropriate fuel source? I did. I spent a lot of time working on my digestion so I could eat all the fat without the side effects I previously had like nausea, cystic acne and itchy skin. If I never took this step and I tried to eat 190+ grams of fat on some days, I. Would. Die. I mean, not literally, but almost. Let's just say it would be a very busy day with many trips to the bathroom.

Carbs

There are days I eat close to 50 grams of carbs and easily stay in ketosis. When I first started, I had to stay closer to 20-30 grams max. Overtime I have become more active and my metabolism has become more flexible. That means I can eat more than 20 carbs in a day and still have the results I want. Is this possible for you? Perhaps, if you work at it. If you are already very active, it may be possible for you today.

While we are on the subject of carbs, I listed both my carb intake and my net carb intake. I personally believe using net carbs is for cheaters. I know not everyone follows my beliefs, so I listed both. If you are going by net carbs because the carbs you are subtracting out are from real foods like vegetables, you can get probably get away with that. If you are subtracting all kinds of strange sugar alcohols and "other carbs" listed on packaged foods that your body doesn't even know how to process in the first place, STOP IT! Now you are a big fat cheater!

I guess if it works for you then do it, but don't say I told you to do it. I very clearly told you to stop that cheater, cheater pumpkin eater behavior above. Eating foods regularly that your body cannot process is only going to lead to storing toxins (fat) and poor health long term.

I used to eat the cheater carbs too. That was in my days of yo-yo diets and not being able to stick with low-carb, high-fat long term because I was not providing my body with real food it was able to digest. Now that I provide my body the good stuff it requires to thrive, this has become a lifestyle. A lifestyle means I will never regain all of the weight I lost after I stop my diet, because I am not on a diet.

Protein

You might also notice my protein intake is sometimes on the higher end of the spectrum for a ketogenic diet. Again, this is the right amount of protein for me to feel good while still getting the results I want. I practice intermittent fasting daily and strength training two to three times per week. The protein and fasting are helping me build the muscle for the results I desire. You may not be able to eat 80-90 grams of protein per day based on your body or goals. Tinker around to see what is right for you. If you don't know where to even start, I am helping people figure this out everyday in my *Coach Me Course.* You could very well be the next person I help!

Back to protein. I could easily lower protein by removing the collagen in my drinks, but collagen is too important for my health. I am steadily approaching 40. Health has become my main goal in place of hitting a number according to macros that are magical to someone else. Collagen provides many health benefits and I am still strumming along in ketosis at 90 grams of protein per day.

Calories

There are rough estimates of calorie counts listed in the daily menus. This is for your benefit, not mine. I gave up calorie counting long ago. I realized counting calories to lose weight was all a big piece of fiction, so I no longer care about calories. I am aware I am the exception to this rule. I am also aware that I have no clue how many calories I take in on a daily basis for the first time in my life, while simultaneously no longer struggling with yo-yoing weight for the first time in my life. There is a connection. Eating to feel good is the connection. There is no connection when you eat to hit a calorie count as designed by an app on your phone. *You* do what you gotta do to get your results.

I also no longer measure my food. I tried to provide general estimates on the foods when I could, but I cannot bring myself back into that tortured mindset any longer. I don't want to steer you in that direction either. I measured, weighed and counted every ounce of food for decades. That only made me insane, while keeping me in fat girl pants.

If measuring and tracking is still your thing, just know I typically eat around 3-4 ounces of meat or 5-6 ounces if the meat is combined with some type of sauce like the sweet & spicy spaghetti sauce. I think. I honestly fill my plate with what I think will satisfy me and stop when I feel good. If I am still hungry, I get more. Since I took the time to improve the way my body digests foods and I eat mostly real food, I don't have to worry about measuring or counting anything beyond a basic guess at carbs.

Day 1
Macros: *Cals:* 2005 *Pro:* 90 *Carbs:* 46 *Net:* 32 *Fat:* 170

10 am
- 1 chocolate protein cupcake
- 1 chocolate butter
- 2 minty melts

12:30 pm
- 2 minty melts
- Bacon avocado & cucumber salad

3 pm
- 2 peanut butter fat bombs
- Handful of walnuts (½ oz)

5:30 pm
- Mediterranean steak strips
- Keto rings
- 2 squares Theo's 85% dark chocolate

Day 2
Macros: *Cals:* 1638 *Pro:* 90 *Carbs:* 38 *Net:* 28 *Fat:* 131

10 am
- BBQ & bruschetta scrambled eggs
- 2 sausages with melted butter on top
- 1 cream cheese fat bomb

12 pm
- Garlic butter chicken (leftovers)
- 4 oz cucumbers drizzled with ranch
- 1 chocolate butter

3 pm
- 1 peanut butter fat bomb
- 1 dark chocolate peanut butter cup
- Handful of almonds (½ oz)

5:30 pm
- Sweet and spicy spaghetti sauce
- 2 squares Theo's dark chocolate

Day 3

Macros: *Cals:* 1865 *Pro:* 89 *Carbs:* 35 *Net:* 20 *Fat:* 157

11 am
- Keto cold buster tea with Perfect Keto collagen

11:20 am
- 2 minty melts
- 1 crumbly PB bar

1 pm
- Mediterranean steak strips (leftovers)
- Spinach salad with walnuts, cucumbers, onions, avocado and ranch
- 2 almond butter bombs

5 pm
- Layered taco salad
- Mexi Caulirice (½ recipe serving)
  Whipped cream with chocolate butter sauce (½ cup whipped)

Day 4

Macros: *Cals:* 2165 *Pro:* 81 *Carbs:* 38 *Net:* 28 *Fat:* 193

10 am
- Salted caramel hot chocolate
- 1 caramel apple fat bomb

12:30 pm
- 4 oz cucumbers drizzled with ranch
- Chicken with Buffalo butter sauce
- 2 minty melts

3 pm
- 1 chocolate pecan ball
- 1 chocolate butter

5:30 pm
- Sausage crust pizza (⅓ recipe)
- 1 peanut butter fat bomb

Day 5
Macros: *Cals:* 1723 *Pro:* 77 *Carbs:* 32 *Net:* 22 *Fat:* 149

12 pm
- The Mac Salad
- 1 chocolate butter
- 1 almond butter bomb

3 pm
- Handful almonds (½ oz)
- 3 minty melts

5:30 pm
- Shredded Chicken Bacon Alfredo
- Spinach salad with walnuts, cucumbers, onions, and ranch
- Garlic butter fried rice (½ recipe serving)
- 2 squares Theo's dark chocolate

Day 6
Macros: *Cals:* 2040 *Pro:* 88 *Carbs:* 29 *Net:* 22 *Fat:* 178

10 am
- Easy scrambled eggs topped with butter
- 4 slices of bacon
- 2 peanut butter fat bombs

12:30 pm
- Keto cold buster tea with Perfect Keto collagen
- 1 crumbly PB bar
- 1 chocolate pecan ball
- 1 minty melt

3 pm
- 4 oz cucumbers drizzled with ranch
- Handful walnuts

5:30 pm
- Buffalo ranch taco salad
- 1 minty melt

Day 7
Macros: *Cals:* 1907 *Pro:* 89 *Carbs:* 34 *Net:* 22 *Fat:* 162

10 am
- Keto cold buster tea with Perfect Keto collagen

10:30 am
- 1 dark chocolate protein cupcake
- 3 minty melts

1 pm
- Chicken avocado salad
- Handful of almonds (½ oz)
- 2 walnut fudge bombs

4 pm
- 1 peanut butter bomb
- 1 cheesecake fat bomb

5:30 pm
- Spicy burger with mayo and mustard
- Coconut sauteed onions (½ recipe serving)
- Creamy garlic green beans (½ recipe serving)
- 1 minty melt

Thank you!

Thank you so much for testing out these delicious recipes I put together this past year. For even more recipes not included in this book, visit my website eatingfatisthenewskinny.com. You will also find plenty more health musings, life lessons and entertaining articles for your viewing pleasure.

If you want to learn more of tips that saved me from a life of desperation and fat girl clothes, read *My Big Fat Life Transformation* on Amazon. I have been blessed to help many people this past year with all of the knowledge I've gained regarding digestion, intermittent fasting and high-fat, low-carb diets. I am excited to spread the high-fat love even further.

If you are ready for all the health knowledge, enroll in my *Coach Me Course: Escape Diet Mentality and End Yo-Yo Diets Forever.* There is waaaaaayyyyyy more to this fabulous lifestyle than move more, eat less...especially since that's not even a real thing! I am teaching students everyday how I *eat more and move less* for better health in my virtual coaching course.

People can scream, "Keto and IF!" at you all day long - but do you even know what in the bologna sandwiches they are talking about? And if you are still eating bologna sandwiches, YOU NEED MY COURSE IN YOUR LIFE NOW!

If you want to take your health progress to the next level, sign up for my *Teach Me Course.* This is the combo package of my six week motivational course combined with the 12 Week Online Fat Loss Course that changed my life forever! You will not find any greater health knowledge out there...especially in a discounted combo deal!

More About Nissa

Graun:

I followed mainstream diet advice for more than twenty five years. I was constantly sick, tired and miserable for the majority of those two plus decades. Sometimes I lost weight, but it was always a difficult process and the weight was routinely gained back within a year, plus more. The chronic illness always remained a constant.

After hitting an all time high weight of 245 pounds after the birth of my first child, I felt completely helpless. All of my previous methods of weight loss were absolutely useless. I was fat, sick, and miserable while still wearing maternity clothes many months after the birth of my first son.

I came across a book and course that changed my life. I learned how to use natural supplements and nutrition to not only take off the weight, but also improve all of the health issues that had been plaguing me longer than I can remember. I set out with intentions of dropping weight that was not budging via any other method, while unintentionally correcting many health problems that afflicted me for decades. These include chronic heartburn, cystic acne, frequent migraines and headaches, frequent sinus infections, constant drippy nose, itchy skin, insomnia, nausea, frequent anxiety, constipation, occasional depression, hypoglycemia, diabetic level blood sugars and constant junk food cravings, just to name a few.

Four years later I am thriving. Keeping the weight off has been a piece of cake. Oh, and I no longer want to eat cake. My weight is now at its lowest point and easily maintained. Now that my digestion is healed and I know the foods that keep me satisfied, living life no longer feels like work. For the first time in my life the constant food noise is gone and I am left with food freedom.

While I have always been passionate about health, I finally know what true health feels like. My passion is to help others achieve their optimal health as well through my blogs, recipes and personal health coaching. Follow me on Instagram or Facebook: @eatingfatisthenewskinny

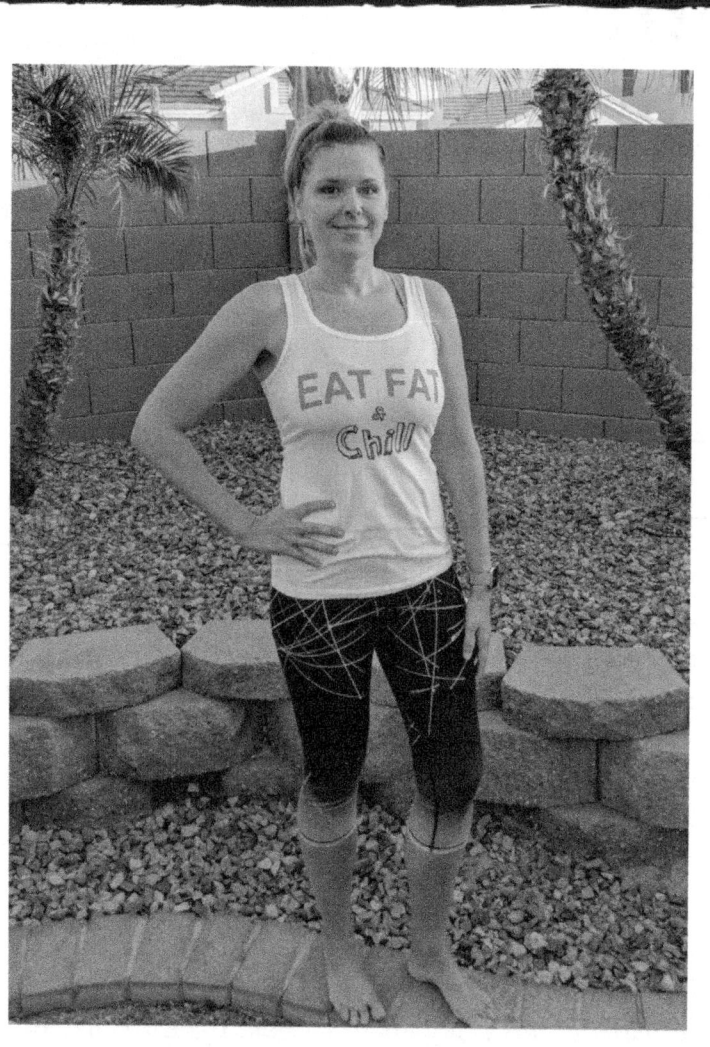